A PHYSICIAN GUIDEBOOK
TO
THE BEST PATIENT EXPERIENCE

A PHYSICIAN GUIDEBOOK

TO

THE BEST PATIENT
EXPERIENCE

BO SNYDER

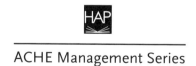

ACHE Management Series

Your board, staff, or clients may also benefit from this book's insight. For more information on quantity discounts, contact the Health Administration Press Marketing Manager at (312) 424-9450.

This publication is intended to provide accurate and authoritative information in regard to the subject matter covered. It is sold, or otherwise provided, with the understanding that the publisher is not engaged in rendering professional services. If professional advice or other expert assistance is required, the services of a competent professional should be sought.

The statements and opinions contained in this book are strictly those of the author and do not represent the official positions of the American College of Healthcare Executives or the Foundation of the American College of Healthcare Executives.

21   20   19   18   17   5   4   3   2   1

Library of Congress Cataloging-in-Publication Data

Names: Snyder, Bo, author.
Title: A physician guidebook to the best patient experience / Bo Snyder.
Description: Chicago, IL : HAP, [2017] | Includes bibliographical references.
Identifiers: LCCN 2016013596 (print) | LCCN 2016021398 (ebook) | ISBN 9781567938319 (print : alk. paper) | ISBN 9781567938333 (xml) | ISBN 9781567938340 (epub) | ISBN 9781567938357 (mobi)
Subjects: LCSH: Patient satisfaction. | Physician and patient. | Interpersonal communication.
Classification: LCC R727.3 .S598 2017 (print) | LCC R727.3 (ebook) | DDC 610.69/6–dc23
LC record available at https://lccn.loc.gov/2016013596

The paper used in this publication meets the minimum requirements of American National Standard for Information Sciences—Permanence of Paper for Printed Library Materials, ANSI Z39.48-1984.♾™

Acquisitions editor: Tulie O'Connor; Manuscript editor: Joyce Dunne; Project manager: Andrew Baumann; Cover designer: Laurie Ingram; Layout: Cepheus Edmondson

Found an error or a typo? We want to know! Please e-mail it to hapbooks@ache.org, mentioning the book's title and putting "Book Error" in the subject line.

For photocopying and copyright information, please contact Copyright Clearance Center at www.copyright.com or at (978) 750-8400.

Health Administration Press
A division of the Foundation of the American
    College of Healthcare Executives
One North Franklin Street, Suite 1700
Chicago, IL 60606-3529
(312) 424-2800

To my wife, Jenny, and daughters, Ellie and Maisie, who've inserted a lot of fun into my life—most of the time in unexpected ways, like introducing (many) new pets to the household without democratic process and giving me a unique "dad" nickname I treasure.

I thank them for their humor and wisdom and, most of all, for their support.

Contents

Preface

I'VE WRITTEN THIS book because I want to help.

The rules of the medical care industry are changing, and doctors increasingly need help in navigating those changes to be successful with the "new normal."

A few decades ago, the quality of a physician's relationship with a patient was judged subjectively—patient by patient. If a relationship was especially good or bad, word of mouth was about the only way anyone else would know.

But now doctors are at the mercy of patient satisfaction surveys (and the reimbursement methodologies tied to those surveys), patients posting their thoughts on Yelp and other Internet ratings sites, and physician performance reporting mandates.

Launched with good intentions and fraught with imperfections, these forces will continue to grow and mature. By the time today's youngest physicians retire, these ways of measuring performance will have evolved into a system that is "just how things are." And the pathway from here to there is already messy.

Some doctors are wired to care deeply about their interactions with patients, while others—although their number is dwindling—believe what the patient thinks of them is unimportant. Perhaps for most doctors, the issue floats in the background—important, yes, but vying with getting the diagnosis right, performing the procedure correctly, being productive, managing interruptions, and otherwise trying to do a good job with every constraint of our modern medical care system meddling in every minute of their day.

I get that.

But in my years of shadowing and coaching doctors, I've seen that most can improve—and can do so rapidly. And the ones who do not, even those who seem eager and engaged as I coach them, failed for specific reasons. The insights about that dichotomy became the driving force behind this book.

So this volume does three important things. First, it gives you—the physician—the basics on what to do during each patient interaction to ensure it's a good one from the patient's perspective. Second, and most important in practical terms, it helps you make the changes necessary to receive better patient satisfaction scores—and make those changes stick. Knowing what to do and consistently doing it are two different concepts. And third, this book outlines ways you can positively influence the organization in which you work so that it will give you and your partners practical, realistic support in this effort.

Congratulations on having the interest and making the time to read this book. It demonstrates motivation, and motivation is a big part of the battle. I hope you'll look back on this book as a turning point in how you relate to patients. Let's get to it!

Bo Snyder

ABOUT THE FIRST VOLUME IN THIS SERIES

My first book on the topic of patients' experience with the healthcare system, *The Best Patient Experience: Helping Physicians Improve Care, Satisfaction, and Scores*, was written for leaders in healthcare organizations. Its goal is to help *them* to help *you* have better interactions with your patients. Although some content of that book is summarized here, you might consider referring your administrator, medical director, or CEO to it.

Acknowledgments

I AM INDEBTED to Dr. Brian Tsang and Lissa Singer at First Physician Corporation (FPC), who allowed their group to serve as the case study presented in Chapter 8. And to everyone at FPC, thank you for your support, for wanting to be the best, and for being role models to provider groups everywhere.

The later chapters (Part V of this book), which offer advice specific to practice settings, were improved with feedback from Dr. Tsang (emergency medicine), Drs. Ana Laus and Jamie Witkowski (hospitalists with insights on the inpatient setting), and Dr. Peter Baldwin (family practice with insights on the office setting).

Many thanks to the talented physicians, physician assistants, and nurse practitioners I have had the pleasure to coach. I've watched these masters of their craft make a huge impact on the lives of their patients—building trust and mutual respect while facing the time constraints imposed by our modern medical system. Just when I think I've seen every trick of the trade, one of you surprises me with something even more incredible that I can share with future clients.

I also want to acknowledge those who have not made as much progress or are still struggling with their interactions with patients. You have prompted me to dig deeper for creative answers and to look more widely for solutions. You're the reason this book is as robust and helpful as I believe it is.

Friends at Arbor Associates—Don Cohen, president, and Larry Willis, CEO—have been sources of much information over the years. Their knowledge of patient satisfaction survey questions and tools is unrivaled, and their insights into ways to use survey data to improve have helped me and my clients tremendously.

Bill Parsons introduced me to *The 4 Disciplines of Execution* (McChesney, Covey, and Huling 2012) and leader standard work—concepts that play an important role both in this book and in the companion volume that shows leaders how they can better support their doctors on this journey. These ideas have helped me improve how I work with clients and changed the way I view leadership.

Finally, I thank my wife, Jennifer Syndergaard Snyder, who was incredibly supportive at every step, beginning with, "Hey, I think you've got enough stuff here to write another book." I—and the editors at Health Administration Press—owe her much for her input on early drafts.

Speaking of the folks at Health Administration Press, they have now helped me publish two books that are much improved from the submitted manuscript but that still let my writing sound like my writing. An author can't ask for anything more.

REFERENCE

McChesney, C., S. Covey, and J. Huling. 2012. *The 4 Disciplines of Execution: Achieving Your Wildly Important Goals*. New York: Free Press.

Introduction

IMAGINE A CONVERSATION among a small group of physicians discussing their poor patient satisfaction scores (or perhaps the fact that they get too many patient complaints).

The medical director says, "We've got to work on this."

To this, Dr. A says, "OK, sure. That would be a good thing to do. Just tell me what to do and I'll do it."

Dr. B says, "Given all the @#$% priorities I have to fit into my day, patient satisfaction is the least of my worries!"

Six months later, which of these physicians is more likely to have made changes? In my experience, *neither* physician is likely to have made much progress. It's not hard to imagine that Dr. B won't address her challenges. But what about Dr. A?

If pressed, I'd say Dr. A has a *slightly* better chance of improving than Dr. B has, but not to much lasting effect. Despite his best intentions, Dr. A is human. And on top of that, he's an incredibly busy human with many different priorities in his professional, not to mention personal, life. His chosen career makes him a very important cog in an incredibly complex, and at times mostly disorganized, system.

And his challenge is daunting: He's being asked to rewire behaviors that have been routine for many years, even decades—behaviors he doesn't even think about anymore.

And on top of all *that*, he doesn't exactly know what he should be doing differently.

HOW CAN DR. A SUCCEED?

Chances are, if you are reading this book, you're more like Dr. A than Dr. B. You have an inkling you could better engage with your patients. Maybe you just received your latest patient satisfaction scores and you don't like what you saw. Or you just received a patient complaint that you have to admit is legitimate.

Or maybe someone has asked you to work on patient satisfaction and handed you this book! (Or maybe you *are* Dr. B, and your medical director told you he's tired of your attitude and you need to improve your scores or find a new job. Ouch! Keep reading.)

Whatever the reason, you're ready to make some changes in your practice routine that will improve your interactions with patients. Great first step.

What's next? From years of coaching physicians, I know that what most of you want is to jump right to a list of behaviors that will improve your interactions with patients. So the book starts with that. But as you read Chapter 1, please keep in mind that I consider Chapter 4 to contain much more important content. It's about *how*, not *what*, to change.

Knowing you need to make changes is not the same as knowing *what* to change, is not the same as knowing *how* to change, and is not the same as knowing how to make a change *stick*.

Chapter 4 lays out a proven process for achieving that first victory. Other victories will follow, and in six months you'll be a different doctor in the eyes of your patients. And of course your patient satisfaction scores will reflect that change as well.

IN A NUTSHELL: A PROVEN METHOD FOR *SUCCESSFUL* BEHAVIOR CHANGE

Because Chapter 4 is so important, I'll give you a preview here. These are the basic steps to hardwiring positive change:

1. Thoughtfully choose one key behavior change (Chapter 1 has many examples) that will have the greatest impact on how much your patients appreciate you.
2. Find a prominent place in your brain to keep track of that one key behavior.
3. Practice that one key behavior with every patient (when it's appropriate) until you do it without thinking. (This shift usually happens in less than a month.)
4. Move on to the next most important behavior change and repeat the process.

This sounds simple, and it is. *But it's not easy*. It could be easy if changing this behavior were the only thing going on in your life. But of course it's not. So to make change manageable, the key is to identify and focus solely on one thing—one small behavior change—at a time.

My experience with hundreds of physicians tells me that making and sustaining behavioral changes takes self-reflection and discipline. You have to seek input from others in intentional ways. (If you're lucky, you'll get dedicated support from your organization. If you don't have that support, I show you in Chapter 7 how to get it from other places or how to go it alone.) And it takes some dedication. You have to keep at it.

The challenge of making lasting behavior change is complex, and it must be addressed from multiple directions. Which brings us to a preview of what you'll find in this book.

WHAT'S IN THIS BOOK

Here is a breakdown, chapter by chapter.

Part I: For Doctors Who Say, "Just Tell Me What to Do and I'll Do It"

As I've said, if you're like most of my coaching clients, this is where instinct tells you to start. Part I includes the following topics:

- The nuts-and-bolts behaviors that add up to great physician–patient interactions are presented in Chapter 1. This content is drawn from the most frequent advice I have given my clients over the years based on my observations of them interacting with patients.
- Chapter 2 focuses on what patients want. It breaks down the questions from patient satisfaction surveys and indicates which behaviors can lead to higher scores on each question. Read this to know "what questions will be on the test."

Part II: How Physicians Can Make and Sustain Behavior Changes

This part of the book is where the real treasure is buried: how to use the information you learned in Part I *to actually alter your behavior*.

- Chapter 3 gives you some background on the science of behavior change. It's a bit academic, but I keep it short and meaningful.
- As mentioned earlier, Chapter 4 provides the most important information in the book: how to make and sustain behavior changes. Using these insights tends to differentiate my successful clients from those who are, let's say, still working on being successful.

Part III: Resources for the Improvement Journey

The tools shared in Part III can support, accelerate, and sustain your efforts to have better interactions with patients.

- The practical resources in Chapter 5 include a self-assessment questionnaire, a worksheet to help you identify where to start, questionnaires for staff and peer feedback, and a sample scorecard and action plan to help you track your progress. Success does not require that you use all, or even any, of these tools, but they have helped others on their journeys.
- Because my most successful clients have organizations that support them, Chapter 6 lists 16 ways that your organization might support you as you look to improve. This list might open your eyes to resources that you can tap—or it may encourage you to ask your organization to make such resources available.
- If you come to the conclusion that you won't get much support from your organization (or if you just need more than it can give you now), Chapter 7 tells you how to go it alone—successfully.
- Chapter 8, the case study, is from one of my most accomplished client groups, which has generously allowed me to use its story. The case illustrates how group support can be useful while demonstrating strategies that can help you make the improvement journey alone. Most important, through its story, this group proves that dramatic improvement can be made in relatively short order.

Part IV: For Skeptics

Even doctors who genuinely want to improve may have reservations about committing to an improvement process. Or maybe you work with physicians who are unconvinced of the importance of patient satisfaction and you need compelling responses when they object to these efforts.

- Chapter 9 covers a dozen reasons doctors should care about patient satisfaction. Some of these will be familiar; others may expand your thinking.
- In Chapter 10, I suggest responses to the most common objections I hear from physicians who don't want to engage on the issue of patient satisfaction.

Part V: Additional Advice Specific to Specialty or Practice Setting

Although physicians across disciplines and settings share many traits and encounter numerous similar challenges, those who practice in certain areas may face additional, unique situations. The specific specialties and settings I address in Part V are

- emergency medicine doctors and urgent care providers (Chapter 11),
- hospitalists or other physicians who round on inpatients (Chapter 12), and
- primary care physicians or other physicians who see patients in an office setting (Chapter 13).

So let's get started. As promised, the book leads off with responses to the perennial request "Just tell me what to do."

Part I

FOR DOCTORS WHO SAY, "JUST TELL ME WHAT TO DO AND I'LL DO IT"

CHAPTER 1

Nuts-and-Bolts Advice for Improving Interactions with Patients

When I shadow and coach physicians, I see the same challenges over and over again. Having meaningful relationships with patients can be an art, but it's also a science. Patient interactions usually follow predictable patterns, and one can dissect and examine those patterns to identify specific behaviors to improve. Even doctors who are naturals at interacting with patients can improve at least a bit by having their eyes opened to a few new opportunities.

I've gathered the insights in this chapter from observing hundreds of physicians *in situ*—interacting with real patients. Here, I break down the patient interactions into a list of practical how-to items. This is the list for those who say, "I want to get better at this. Tell me what I need to do."

Is this you? If so, you're already interested and engaged. If you are also disciplined and follow through, you will be able to move the needle on your patient satisfaction scores a long way in the right direction in a short period of time.

THE DETAILS

In the following sections, I describe the most common opportunities for improvement I've identified for physicians interacting with patients (summarized in Exhibit 1.1). These opportunities have to do with awareness, first impressions, the phase I call "the meaty middle," and last impressions.

These practical tips are effective and easy to implement—if you master them one at a time, as demonstrated in Chapter 4. I offer them as a means to structure your analysis of your own performance—what you already do with your patients and opportunities you may not have considered before.

Exhibit 1.1: A Framework for Engaging Patients

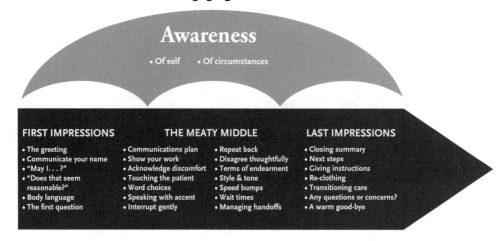

Awareness
- Of self
- Of circumstances

FIRST IMPRESSIONS	THE MEATY MIDDLE		LAST IMPRESSIONS
• The greeting	• Communications plan	• Repeat back	• Closing summary
• Communicate your name	• Show your work	• Disagree thoughtfully	• Next steps
• "May I. . . ?"	• Acknowledge discomfort	• Terms of endearment	• Giving instructions
• "Does that seem reasonable?"	• Touching the patient	• Style & tone	• Re-clothing
• Body language	• Word choices	• Speed bumps	• Transitioning care
• The first question	• Speaking with accent	• Wait times	• Any questions or concerns?
	• Interrupt gently	• Managing handoffs	• A warm good-bye

Source: Adapted from Snyder (2016).

Awareness: The Tip That Tops All Others

No aspect of your performance is more important to your success than being aware that your interaction with the patient is very important. This consciousness places you in a frame of mind to win her confidence and make her feel fortunate that she has you as her doctor.

Awareness allows you to remind yourself before each encounter to consider what your patient might be thinking and likely is experiencing. See yourself as a helping partner, not just a clinical decision maker.

Over the years, I've watched many doctors improve their patient satisfaction scores before they analyze a single micro-aspect of their patient interactions. In fact, most doctors can improve their scores by simply stepping into the right state of mind before every interaction. And by the way, this is why doctors who are just naturally good with patients are that way—they're continually mindful of it.

This "right state of mind" includes paying attention to your sixth sense—your ability to perceive or intuit what is going on in certain interactions or circumstances. And yes, you do have this ability. Did your medical training teach it to you? Probably not, but your experience as a human being tells you it's real. Pay attention to it.

It's one thing to tell yourself, "With each patient today, I will pause and remind myself to be aware"—of yourself, the patient's needs, the immediate circumstances, and what that patient will reflect back on when he fills out his patient satisfaction survey or when he tells his bowling buddies about you. It's another thing to do it prior to each and every encounter. Practice the following tips until the approach becomes second nature:

- Before seeing a patient, pause and say to yourself, *"I am going to care for this patient like he is a member of my family."*
- Apply the principle behind the expression *"The best judge of character is how someone treats a waiter when no one is watching."* Pretend that your patient satisfaction coach—or better yet, the person responsible for renewing your contract—is monitoring you and taking notes. Or that your aunt (who thinks you walk on water) is watching. Don't disappoint her!
- Finally, understand that, in essence, you *are* always being observed: The patient satisfaction survey is always "watching."

This list is a general approach to being aware. Following is a discussion of specific types of awareness to practice in your patient encounters.

Self-Awareness

Feeling tired? Dealing with a difficult patient? Time to be on guard.

By being self-aware, you can often predict when you're headed for rough waters. Know your triggers—everyone has them. Then institute the following tips to make potentially stressful encounters go more smoothly:

- Before you see a patient who has been challenging in the past, say to yourself, *"I know I could easily get snippy with this patient. I won't do that. I'm the professional in the conversation. I will not take the bait. I will not let this be the* one *patient who torpedoes my patient satisfaction scores this month."*
- Take a deep breath in the middle of the conversation. Focus on being very controlled in your responses, being mindful of your triggers. Be gentle and strong at the same time.
- If a patient challenges a mistake by a colleague (your partner who rounded yesterday in your place, for example), don't feel the need to be defensive. Just move ahead with what you can do to help that patient today.

Awareness of Circumstances: When You're Out-of-Control Busy

Doctors tell me the biggest barrier to better patient satisfaction is not having enough time to spend with their patients because of their workload. I empathize with this—and don't have an easy answer. I know that most doctors struggle with this issue to varying degrees. However, I've worked with many doctors who have earned high patient satisfaction scores in spite of it.

***The Broad View of Improving Patient Interactions: Three Key Concepts
and One Important Truth***

This chapter might seem to cover more tips than anyone can implement.
Don't panic! Ease into this process by thinking about the three concepts
introduced below. If these are all you take away from this chapter, you'll still
be on your way to improving your patient encounters.

1. *Be aware.* Prior to every patient interaction, remind yourself of its
   importance. Prepare to be "on." Pause before entering the room
   to collect yourself and focus on having a great exchange with the
   patient. Pay attention when intuition tells you to.

   Just being aware helps many doctors make small—even
   subconscious—adjustments in the way they interact with patients.

2. *Make a great first impression.* Knock and ask permission before
   entering. Say hello and introduce yourself. Tell your patient you've
   read her chart, but you'd like to hear what brought her in today (or, if
   she's an inpatient, how she feels today).

   The point is to take a moment to establish a relationship and hear
   the patient's story before diving into "the doctor thing."

3. *Make a great last impression.* Summarize the main points both you
   and the patient have communicated. Cover next steps. Ask if he has
   any unanswered questions. Offer a warm goodbye.

   The key idea here is to pause and take your time wrapping up the
   meeting. Make sure the patient is comfortable with everything you've
   covered before you leave the room.

Now, let's say you want to dive a little deeper. My one important truth is this:

> *Memorizing my list of tips won't be helpful for most doctors.*

Trying to tweak every aspect of your routine with patients will be
overwhelming and counterproductive. Trying to do too many things
differently all at once will throw anyone off his game.

Instead, scan the tips and decide which presents *your* biggest opportunity
to make *one* change that will have significant impact.

If you need some guidance on which to choose, feel free to jump ahead
and (1) complete a self-assessment (see Appendix 5.1 on pages 60–62);

(continued)

(continued from previous page)

(2) ask your physician colleagues, a nurse, or a medical assistant to observe you with patients and provide feedback (see Appendix 5.3 on pages 64–66); (3) work with a professional coach; or (4) rank-order your opportunities for improvement to pinpoint the one that will yield the most improvement (see Appendix 5.2 on page 63).

As described in detail later in the book, work on making only that one change. Keep at it until you have mastered it and it has become a natural part of your routine. Rewiring a brain can take several weeks or a month, so don't give up after only a few tries.

Once your first priority has been mastered, move on to your second-most-impactful opportunity. And repeat from there. Slowly mastering key changes based on your individual strengths and weaknesses will have a significant and lasting impact on your patients' satisfaction for the rest of your career.

Especially when your workload is incredibly high, I advise this: Your goal—as the professional—is to not let your patient *see* how busy you are.

Patients get anxious if they can tell that your workload is excessive. So remember the adage "Never let 'em see you sweat." Before you enter the room, say to yourself:

My job is to not let the patient see how crazy this day is for me. I will not use that as an excuse. I will not let that cause my patient any anxiety. I'm taking a deep breath and not letting my crazy day affect this patient's experience. I will not let my body language betray me. It's my job to protect this patient from the harried realities of the modern healthcare system.

There is no magic answer, but your best efforts to keep your wits on those super-hectic days are often noticed by your patients.

When you really can't spend much time, concentrate on giving the patient a great few minutes. Be fully present, and make sure you end the interaction positively. Ask for questions, even if you don't believe you have much time to answer. Ask if there's anything else you can do for the patient.

Remember that needing to get out of the room to see your next patient is different from *seeming* like you *want* to get out of the room to see your next patient. Your patients know you're busy. Don't underscore the point by checking your pager or forgetting to say goodbye. As discussed in detail in a later section, don't let your body language betray you.

First Impressions

Get the interaction off to a good start with each patient. It's crucial: The old adage about not getting a second chance to make a first impression is never more true than in your exam room. With the tips that follow, you can start building a relationship of communication and trust right away.

The Greeting

Begin an interaction with a patient—especially a new one—by knocking on the door, introducing yourself by name, stating that you are his doctor today, and shaking his hand, if appropriate.

Give the patient your full attention during the greeting. Maintain eye contact, and don't try to multitask. For example, instead of turning your back to the patient during your introduction to pull gloves out of a box on the wall, separate your actions with a phrase such as, *"Let me put on my gloves before we talk further. I want to give you my full attention."*

If the patient is an inpatient, ask if this is a good time to talk with him, perhaps saying, *"May I come in now to talk with you?"* In addition to being courteous, this question gives the patient some feeling of control (more on this later in the chapter).

Close the door or curtain for privacy—and tell the patient that's why you're doing it, so he gives you credit for it. In an inpatient setting, ask for permission to adjust the volume of the television: *"May I turn the TV volume off so we can hear each other better?"* Many physicians turn down the volume without asking. While their instincts are good, they are infringing on the patient's space without permission *and* they've just missed an opportunity to build the relationship.

Give Them Ways to Remember Your Name

Make sure your lab coat displays your name clearly in letters that are large and easy to read (no cursive). Anxious patients and family members often will not remember your name from your verbal introduction, or remember it accurately, if your name is more exotic than (or as common as) Smith or Jones. So make it easy for them to sneak a peek at your lab coat during the visit to see your name and cement it in their memory. This is information they want and need. If you're also wearing a name badge, so much the better. Affix the badge firmly so that it doesn't flip over backward.

Strongly consider using business cards. Some doctors have their pictures on their cards, which is incredibly helpful for patients and families. It will be hard for the patient to remember your name when you've just met for the first time, especially if the patient sees more than one doctor. A business card left at the close of a first interaction will make sure your patient has your name and a way to follow up with you if needed. It's a thoughtful gesture to wrap up with.

Do You Have an Achilles Heel?

Sometimes when I shadow physicians with middling patient satisfaction scores, I don't see any huge problems. But just when I start wondering why their scores aren't higher, I notice a single *something*. The issue might not arise with every patient, but it isn't long before I see it again—and then again.

The Achilles heel—that one big flaw that doctors don't recognize—tends to dilute their otherwise excellent performance. But once they fix the flaw, they become patient satisfaction superstars.

Some classic Achilles heel behaviors I've encountered in physicians include the following:

- Checking their watch or pager while the patient is talking
- Interrupting when the patient is trying to answer their questions
- Arguing with the patient (about anything)
- Excusing themselves from the room before they have answered all the patient's questions
- Speaking critically of other members of the care team, even if that criticism is deserved

Do you have an Achilles heel? How can you know? Follow the steps discussed in the previous sidebar in this chapter (pages 6–7). And you should also look at the verbatim comments your patients have given to the open-ended questions on your patient satisfaction survey.

Once you've found your Achilles heel, resolve to fix it—just it—no matter if you've discovered other little things you should change. Save those for later. For now, zero in on your single most patient-annoying behavior.

Tell your staff and your partners what you're working on. Sharing this information will make you feel more accountable for sticking with it.

Give Patients More Control: Two Magic Phrases

When patients feel they have more control, they will be more satisfied with their overall experience. Especially important at the beginning of the visit is using the words *"May I…"* to ask patients' permission before taking even mundane actions. The opportunity to grant permission gives them control and is likely to increase their respect for you. Opportunities to use these words early on in the visit include the following:

- Before entering her room: *"Good morning, Mrs. Smith. May I come in and talk with you now?"*
- Before beginning a physical examination: *"May I examine you now?"* (Often patients reply, "Why, of course. You're the doctor." If this happens, you can deliver the super-impactful, relationship-building statement, *"No patient has ever told me 'no,' but I always ask before touching a patient. It's your body, and doctors need to respect that."*)

Another way to give the patient control is to always ask, *"Does that seem reasonable?"* when recommending a test or course of treatment. Using this phrase leaves no doubt that the patient has been invited to participate in—and has assumed a measure of control over—her care.

Body Language and Positioning

To sit or not to sit. If your style is more businesslike and formal, or if you tend to move quickly on rounds, consider sitting on the side of the bed or pulling up a chair before beginning the substantive part of the conversation with your patient.

Some folks in our field prescribe sitting because it "forces" the physician to take the time to thoroughly communicate with the patient. I think the value of this advice is overstated. Many physicians are just fine standing; others need to sit to make a better connection. Use your sixth sense or get input from others to figure out which type you are.

Once you know your style, keep in mind the following guidelines for body language and physical positioning:

- If you stand, take care to not overpower the patient with your presence. Stand upright; don't hover over her if you're just talking. Most patients are uncomfortable when their physician stands too close, especially if you are tall. Be careful to stay in a spot where the patient can see you without effort. And if that isn't possible, give her permission to not look at you while you're talking. She'll give you credit for acknowledging her discomfort.

- Be conscious when you first meet a patient to not put your hands on your hips or lean forward too far. Similarly, avoid crossing your arms over your chest. Just drop those arms to your side and relax. "Talking with your hands" is OK, too, if it's natural for you. This aspect of body language is just as important as being still; quelling your natural inclinations to gesture can be distracting.

- Maintain eye contact.

- Laugh and smile when it feels appropriate. If you have a playful side, don't be afraid to let it show when your instincts tell you it's OK. But if the patient doesn't naturally respond to your humor, go back to being polite and professional.

The First Question

Especially if your style is more formal and businesslike, I recommend opening the interaction (after the initial greeting) with a simple open-ended question, such as *"How are you feeling today?"* or *"Are you feeling any differently than you did when we talked yesterday? Can you tell me about it?"*

If you're in an office, urgent care, or emergency department setting, you may start with, *"I've read your chart, but I'd like to hear from you what brought you in today."*

This approach gives the patient a chance to "tell his story" before you begin with any questions or updates. Not being listened to by the doctor is a major dissatisfier for patients. Importantly, as the patient is updating you, fight the urge to interrupt. You can ask follow-up questions later. For now, be an active listener.

For the special cases where the patient might as well be reciting *War and Peace,* with no apparent connection to the situation (what these patients really need is a friend instead of a healthcare provider), do feel free to interrupt. But interrupt as gently as you can: *"What else can you tell me that might help me address [the medical condition]?"* or *"I'm very interested in [something he has already told you]."* Then ask a follow-up question about it.

In any case, don't look at your pager. Don't even check your watch. (Maybe you're old enough to remember when the first President George Bush checked his watch while Bill Clinton was talking during the 1992 presidential debate. The message sent was "I can't wait for this thing to be over!")

If your style is to ask patients questions in rapid-fire fashion, give them a little warning, especially when meeting for the first time. You might say, *"May I ask you some questions to help me assess your situation?"* Then you can jump into questions that delve deeper—and do this in your natural style.

Notice that my suggestion is *not* to slow down your questioning. By giving a little warning first, you'll find that patients won't react negatively to rapid questioning. Consider this notice another opportunity to ask the patient's permission.

If you are extremely extroverted, make sure your personality doesn't overpower a patient when you first meet. Introduce yourself and ask your first questions gently. Once the patient has warmed up and knows your style, you can be more fully yourself.

The Meaty Middle

The steps discussed next will help you ease your patients through the complex essentials of the visit while continuing to connect with them.

Have a Communications Game Plan

If you tend to think in a nonlinear style (or if your patient is easily sidetracked or has proven she can easily sidetrack you), have a go-to game plan for communication throughout the interaction. I suggest the classic three-step process:

1. Tell the patient what you're going to cover.
2. Cover it.
3. Tell the patient what you just covered.

This approach will greatly improve not only the communication itself but also the patient's perception of it—and your resulting patient satisfaction score.

First, once you have greeted the patient, set the agenda for the visit. A hospitalist might say, *"I'd like us to cover three things: I'd like to hear how you're doing today, update you on the results of your tests, and then discuss next steps. I also want to make sure all your questions are answered."* Second, follow the structure you've established in step 1. It will help the patient make sense of the communication. Third, at the end of the interaction, summarize what you covered. The patient will then have heard the information three times and will be more likely to retain it—and give you credit for fantastic communication skills when she fills out the satisfaction survey.

Show Your Work

As you speak with a patient, always explain "why." This helps patients "see you think" as you process information to help them. For patients, medicine is scary, mysterious—a great unknown. They will appreciate having the dots connected.

Remember your eighth-grade math tests, when you had to show how you solved the problem in order to get full credit? Same principle applies here.

As you're examining the patient, share your observations out loud. Even basic feedback such as *"Your lungs sound clear"* will be appreciated. Patients take the physical exam very seriously.

Be sure to explain what you're trying to find out by ordering certain tests. Explain whether a particular result is favorable or unfavorable to them and, most important, what you think about it as a physician. Patients want to see and hear you justify the test and then process the results.

Patients who observe you processing the information while you're sharing it increase their assessment of your credibility and their appreciation of you, as well as their understanding of the situation. The same logic applies when there are choices to be made in next steps. Patients need you to explain why one path is better than another.

Explaining why is especially important if the patient disagrees with you or shows any sign of confusion. In a later section, we discuss handling disagreements specifically.

Acknowledge Discomfort

If you have to move a patient and it causes discomfort, say something like, *"I'm sorry this is causing you pain. But I have to move you to complete your exam. I'll make it as quick as I can. Then we'll try to help you with the pain if it continues."*

On Touching the Patient

If you need to touch a patient in any way that would not be acceptable in a social setting, always give him warning and, ideally, ask permission: *"May I examine you now?"* This demonstration of respect will be noted, appreciated—and remembered.

Speaking and Word Choice

Be conscious of using clinical language. I've heard physicians use *colonization, febrile,* and other terms most patients won't understand. It's impossible to eliminate medical jargon entirely, but be mindful of it. If you catch yourself using such vocabulary, you can recover (and get bonus points) by saying, *"Forgive me for using a clinical term. Let me find a better word."*

If You Speak with an Accent

Recognize that some patients *will* have trouble understanding you and that it's your job to address this challenge. It is not their job to figure out what you said.

Following are some tips to set you both at ease in the interaction:

- Address the issue right up front, and give the patient permission to ask you to repeat yourself: *"You may have guessed that I did not grow up speaking English! Communication is vital to taking good care of you, so please don't feel uncomfortable asking me to repeat anything. I won't be bothered or insulted. I'm used to it!"*

- When a patient can't understand a specific word, don't repeat it. Use a synonym instead. After a while, you will be able to anticipate and avoid such words.
- Speak slowly.
- Make eye contact with the patient whenever you're speaking.
- Don't mistake nodding and smiling for understanding. Often, in fact, it signals the opposite.
- Draw pictures or talk with your hands to help explain.
- Ask a staff member who speaks English as her primary language to be involved in lengthy or high-stakes explanations.
- Rely more on written communications, and to alleviate communication anxieties, let patients know that they will be receiving instructions in writing.
- Use your sense of humor and natural warmth to strengthen the bond with your patient. This approach helps compensate for any communication issues. Instead of being "the doctor I can't understand," be "the doctor I love who happens to speak with an accent."

Interrupt Gently

As discussed earlier in the context of the first question in the encounter, fight the urge to interrupt the patient during the meaty middle of the interaction. It's tempting to jump in when he's going on and on with information that seems to add little value. Instead, look for an opportunity to gently interject, *"I see."* Then ask your redirecting question. To find out what feels most natural to you in these situations, experiment with different ways to regain control of the discussion.

Repeat Back

Demonstrate that you're listening by saying something like, *"This is what I'm hearing you say. . . ."* This may seem corny, but it shows that you really *were* listening, especially after the patient has given a long, involved description.

Not to be overlooked is the need to demonstrate that you're listening by actually listening! Let your patient see you process the information she's given you.

Disagree Thoughtfully

Never argue with a patient. There will be times when you and a patient (or his family) are not in agreement. It's helpful to remember that the patient will ultimately do what he wants to do. It's his life. You may think you can win an argument with a patient, but you never really will.

That said, when you and a patient do disagree, try this process:

1. Let the patient express his point of view. Your job is to quietly listen to every word he says and completely understand where he's coming from, even if it's left field.

2. Say something like, *"I think I know where you're coming from. Let me summarize what I've heard you say."* When you repeat it back, the patient will recognize that you've heard him. This is very important because it shows you are being objective even when you disagree.

3. Present your alternative point of view.

4. Discuss the patient's point of view again, and let him know that you're weighing both perspectives but you think yours has more merit (if, indeed, you still feel that way).

5. See if you can get the patient to also weigh both points of view.

In these types of conversations, avoid the word *can't*—as in, "I can't do that for you." Try to steer the conversation back to what you *can* do. As a last resort, mention that what the patient is requesting *"is something most doctors in this community just don't do."* You're deflecting your unwillingness to take the patient's preferred action onto the profession, and that's just fine if you've exhausted your discussion points.

A special area in which physicians are obliged to disagree is in the case of drug-seeking patients, who show up most often for emergency medicine doctors and hospitalists. I recommend adopting a kind demeanor that is also direct:

> My concern is that those drugs are very addictive and they could easily harm you. But I'd like to refer you to a pain specialist who can help you with your discomfort.

Most drug seekers don't want to have anything to do with a pain specialist, and they tend to know you're onto them when you suggest this.

Because dealing with drug seekers is such a difficult and pervasive issue, I often advise clients to brainstorm best-practice responses to be used by all providers in their group.

I am amazed by some of my clients' masterful dealings with difficult patients. They manage to be strong and gentle at the same time. You can take a tough stand with a patient while also letting her see that you care about her.

The key is to recognize when one of these situations is developing, pause, and say to yourself, *"I can be firm* and *gentle here. My motivation is the patient's best interests, and I will work hard for her to see that."*

With the communication methods outlined in this section, you're modeling exactly how you want the patient to process the issue: calmly and objectively.

Remember, the goal is to get the patient to consider your point of view (not for you to win an argument) so that she is more likely to buy into and comply with your recommended course of treatment.

No Terms of Endearment

If you use the term *dear* with a patient, you'd better be treating a hooved mammal with antlers. Professionals should not use terms of endearment with patients—ever.

The rule on what to call a patient is to use the conservative approach until he gives you permission to do otherwise. "Good morning, Mr. Smith, I'm Dr. Robertson" will never get you in trouble. If your sixth sense tells you the patient is turned off by this degree of formality (by the way, great job using your sixth sense!), then just ask what he'd like you to call him. Most patients appreciate being asked, and it gives them more control in a situation that can be unnerving for them.

Style and Tone

If you tend to be very businesslike and direct, pay attention when intuition tells you to soften your style around certain patients—especially those who seem introverted. Introduce yourself more passively and incorporate pauses to let them speak. Try not to interrupt.

In general, be conservative with your sense of humor. More specifically, use humor when it fits the situation (and suits your personality). Sometimes patients will invite it or reciprocate. If you offer a bit of humor and the patient doesn't respond, don't keep trying. Back away from using it again.

Speed Bumps

As mentioned earlier in the chapter, some doctors are wired for speed—you move fast, you talk fast. Remember that this trait can be viewed negatively by your patient. It sends the message that "My next patient is more important than you are."

To offset a speedy nature, try a slightly slower and more relaxed introduction— especially when you're busy. If you have to move quickly, at least you'll have a better chance of building a connection with the patient if you slow down as you greet him. Then you can return to your normal speed.

You can also try building in some speed bumps by using the techniques suggested earlier in the "Awareness of Circumstances" section:

- Seek permission to ask questions.
- Ask for the go-ahead to perform the physical exam.

- Pause before leaving the room to make sure the patient has no questions. After the patient replies, walk slowly out of the room (you can shift to a trot once you're out of sight).

Related to this last point, you may compensate for how fast you speak by saying something like this at the end of an interaction: *"I know I sometimes talk really fast, so let me pause here to let you ask questions. Was anything unclear?"*

On Wait Times

Often, you can't speed up the process, but you can address patients' uncertainty about wait times. When possible, give them a sense of how long their wait *may* be for a test result or the next step in the care process.

Sometimes you might simply have to say that the wait may be long, and you can't accurately estimate—you don't want to overpromise and end up underdelivering. But even this gesture is helpful to patients because it shows that you are aware and care, and it helps them recalibrate their expectations.

When a patient has been waiting a long time to see you, address the situation head-on using the AAA approach:

Acknowledge

Apologize

Amend

Here's an example:

> I know we've kept you waiting a very long time. I don't like it when my patients have to wait like you have *(acknowledge)*. I want to apologize for your wait—I'm very sorry *(apologize)*. You have my full attention now *(amend)*. What brings you in to the emergency department today?

For more on addressing wait times in the emergency department (ED), see Chapter 11.

Managing Handoffs

Care transitions from one provider or setting to another can cause great upheaval for patients, as when a patient in the ED needs to be admitted. This situation presents patient engagement opportunities for both the emergency medicine physician and the hospitalist. Refer to Chapters 11 and 12 for specific guidance on enhancing physician–patient interactions in ED and inpatient settings.

Last Impressions

Concluding the interaction with clear communication strengthens compliance with your treatment regimen and your relationship with the patient. Using the following approaches at the end of patient encounters can go a long way toward achieving these important goals.

The Closing Summary

I suggest that doctors wrap up most patient interactions by summarizing the key points of the discussion—major test findings and the implications for the patient, next steps, and what those steps mean for the patient. Although you will have already covered this information, the patient needs to hear it again to retain it and act on it.

Remember to continue communicating that the patient has control: *"May we do a brief summary before I leave?"* You're asking permission *and* you're reviewing material with the patient's assistance so that she is more likely to fully understand. Taking these steps also reminds the patient that you listened to her:

> Let me summarize what we covered: I heard you tell me that you're feeling _____ today. Your test results are improving (etc.), and we've got a _____ test scheduled for tomorrow morning. If the result of that test is OK, there's a good chance you can go home tomorrow afternoon.

Remember to ask, *"Does that seem reasonable?"* when making treatment recommendations. This invites the patient to participate in and control her own care.

After your summary, ask if the patient has any more questions. This helps the patient remember what you've told her and improves her perception of your communication skills.

Giving Instructions

Many patient–physician interactions, especially in the ED or in urgent care, conclude with some sort of follow-up instructions. Patients immediately get anxious because they think they have to remember everything you say; they don't realize that they'll hear it all again from your nurse, medical assistant, or care coordinator and then get it in writing.

Preempt this anxiety by making a statement such as this:

> Let me run through what I'd like you to do after you leave today, but don't worry about remembering everything. The nurse will cover it with you again, and then you'll also get instructions in writing to take home. I'm sharing this information with you first to make sure you understand and so that I can answer any questions you might have.

Re-clothing

This advice is specific to office-based doctors: When you're getting ready to leave a patient after examining him, let him know whether he can put his clothes back on. Don't make him wait for the nurse to tell him to get dressed. Patients want to put their clothes back on ASAP, and you'll score extra points when you give them permission to go ahead and do it. You'll turn the room over more quickly, too, which might help your busy schedule.

Transitioning Care

For hospitalists, emergency medicine physicians, and any other physicians who work a shift and need to transition care to another member of the group, refer to the doctor who will follow you as your *partner* or *colleague*. This gives a better impression than saying "another doctor" will be taking over.

The terms *partner* and *colleague* imply that you know and trust the other doctor, which will give the next physician a head start in building a relationship with the patient. The patient will feel more confident knowing she is being cared for by a cohesive team whose members collaborate and communicate.

The Last Question

When appropriate, before you leave—even before you put your hand on that doorknob or curtain—ask whether the patient has any more questions. Consider saying something like, *"Is there anything else that we should cover?"* Pausing to give the patient a moment to think about it shows him your question is sincere.

This type of question is powerful in that it will improve the patient's rating of your communication and your willingness to engage with him. The way you phrase the question can vary; here are some other options:

Do you have any questions I can cover before we wrap up?

Anything else before I go?

Do you have any other concerns we can talk about before I go?

Does everything we've talked about make sense?

And once this portion of the conversation is over, be sure to tell the patient specifically how to follow up with you if he has a question or need later.

A particular piece of advice for hospitalists and other physicians in the inpatient setting is to get into the practice of leaving your business card, especially if patients or family members have asked lots of questions. They will be comforted in knowing they have the means to find you if they need more information.

Some doctors offer their card when they introduce themselves, but I think it has more impact as you're saying goodbye at the end of the first meeting: *"Here's my card; please contact me if you have any questions."*

Finally, rely on your experience and sixth sense to detect whether any issues are lingering that the patient hasn't raised. Patients don't ask questions for many reasons. One is that they want to be respectful of your time. However, it's your job to help patients overcome their own reluctance to raise issues or questions that could be important.

A Warm Goodbye

Always say goodbye to the patient. This gesture signals a positive, formal closure to your interaction, leaving no doubt that you have finished your exchange.

Many physicians miss this opportunity, especially in emergency medicine, and it's usually unintentional: The doctor leaves the room to begin his next task, and the next thing the patient knows, the nurse is coming in with directions to the checkout desk! Believe me, the patient notices your absence every time.

Your intention to return, or not return, must be made clear. If you haven't given a warm goodbye, check in with the patient that one last time. You'll be sending a powerful message: *"I care. So I wouldn't let you go without saying goodbye."*

This goes for office-based physicians, emergency medicine physicians, and urgent care providers, especially. For example, an emergency physician can say,

> I probably won't see you again before you're admitted upstairs. So I wanted to say goodbye and wish you well. I've enjoyed meeting you. I wish it could have been under better circumstances.

There are many ways to say goodbye, including a simple *"I wish you well."* The wording doesn't matter as much as the effort does.

It's often appropriate to end the conversation with a handshake, a squeeze of the hand, or a gentle touch to the shoulder, but only if it feels comfortable to do so.

A NOTE ABOUT SCRIPTING

In this chapter, I offer examples of *situational scripting* to address specific circumstances you will likely encounter: "When X happens, say something similar to Y."

Of course, no patient wants to experience a visit with her doctor that feels forced, impersonal, or insincere. Each interaction is unique, and you will use your professional discretion and common sense to tailor your communication.

That said, some doctors find it helpful to develop specific wording to use in certain situations. Consider all the times in your life that you respond to specific situations with words your brain has scripted. Do you answer the phone the same way every time? Probably.

If you feel the need to self-script with specific words, by all means, do so. Just give yourself permission to change it up a bit if conversations with patients start to feel robotic.

YOU'RE ON YOUR WAY!

Remember, the overarching goal is to increase your *awareness* of how you interact with patients. You can improve your patient satisfaction scores merely by becoming more aware of how you engage with patients.

Becoming practiced at the tools and techniques presented here—one at a time (see Chapter 4)—will accelerate that improvement. Eventually, you will have comfortably incorporated many of these adjustments into your routine—to be pulled out and used when practical and applicable.

Congratulations! Just by reading this chapter, you're already on your way to building better relationships with your patients. Higher patient satisfaction scores won't be far behind.

REFERENCE

Snyder, B. 2016. *The Best Patient Experience: Helping Physicians Improve Care, Satisfaction, and Scores.* Chicago: Health Administration Press.

What Patients Want (Or, It Helps to Know the Questions Before You Take the Test)

"WHAT DO PATIENTS want from me?" It's a question doctors often ask me. While the specifics vary from patient to patient, in general I've found that patients want

a trusting relationship with a skilled, well-mannered
professional who is fully committed to helping them.

This observation is validated by the questions survey vendors use. Although they vary somewhat among vendors, patient satisfaction survey questions tend to be built around the following themes in physician behaviors:

- Exhibiting courtesy and respect
- Listening carefully
- Explaining things in a way patients can understand
- Showing respect for what patients have to say
- Spending enough time with patients
- Giving information about patients' treatment
- Showing concern for patients' comfort
- Including patients in their own care
- Being friendly
- Inspiring faith in the provider's clinical abilities

Many of these themes are interrelated. For example, listening carefully is key to exhibiting courtesy and respect. Providing treatment information and explaining it clearly helps the physician establish credibility in her clinical abilities.

Patient Dissatisfiers

It's helpful to look at the flip side of the patient satisfaction coin—dissatisfaction. Don Cohen, whose company, Arbor Associates, has 30 years' experience collecting and reporting patient satisfaction survey data, shares his organization's survey questions that track patient dissatisfiers.

At the Hospital

Not surprisingly, interaction with providers lies at the heart of patient dissatisfaction in both inpatient and outpatient settings.

Leading inpatient dissatisfiers:

- Not included in care, but wanted to be.
- Nurses did not listen carefully.
- In pain; staff not helpful.
- Doctors did not listen carefully.
- Nurses not friendly.

Leading outpatient dissatisfiers:

- Not included in care, but wanted to be.
- Discharge process deficient (typically due to time limitations). (Note that this is the only dissatisfier unrelated to personal interaction issues.)
- Not made to feel special.
- Doctors not friendly.
- Doctors did not seem skilled (most often noted in the emergency department).

Although several of these points of unhappiness relate to nursing or the overall patient experience, physicians play an important role—directly or indirectly—in many.

Furthermore, because the doctor may see the patient only once a day, the significance of the doctor's role is amplified in a short period of "high stakes" interaction. So not only is patient satisfaction important, but opportunities to achieve it (or compromise it) come at doctors with now-or-never urgency.

(continued)

(continued from previous page)

In the Office

The impact of the doctor is even more important in the office setting, where the leading dissatisfiers are as follows:

- Doctor did not show respect for what I had to say.
- Doctor never or only sometimes knew my medical history.
- Doctor never or only sometimes listened carefully.
- Doctor did not explain things in an easy-to-understand way.
- Patient was not included in care, but wanted to be.

These drivers of patient satisfaction don't let the front-desk staff off the hook for treating patients right. But clearly, the doctor is the main attraction (or—unfortunately—detraction) in the office setting.

Source: D. Cohen, personal communication, March 10, 2014.

Let's take a closer look at each theme and identify some of the physician behaviors from Chapter 1 that best address it.

EXHIBITING COURTESY AND RESPECT

This behavior is nonnegotiable. Showing exceptional courtesy and respect won't boost the scores of an average-scoring doctor, but *not* doing it will drop that doctor closer to the bottom. In other words, patients expect an appropriate degree of courtesy and respect. If they don't get it, they notice.

Every tip in this chapter ultimately affects a patient's perception of courtesy and respect, but let's focus on the basics here:

- Don't seem rushed. Appearing hurried introduces anxiety into the interaction and creates the perception that you might be cutting corners. Keeping a brisk pace is OK, but don't cross the line to looking like you have more important things to do.
- Give the patient your full attention. Repeat to yourself a thousand times, *"I will not check my pager until I leave the room."*
- Make eye contact.
- Greet the patient by name.

- Introduce yourself.
- Shake hands, if appropriate.
- Say goodbye and wish the patient well.

Many of these tips belong in the "everything important I learned in kindergarten" file. If you have any doubts as to whether you're performing these actions consistently, ask those who work with you for feedback and check the verbatim feedback from your patient satisfaction surveys.

LISTENING CAREFULLY

Of course you know that listening carefully is important to providing good care. Otherwise, you might miss information that could influence your clinical decision making.

But do patients *perceive* that you're listening carefully? That's equally important. Following are two tips to ensure that patients view you as attentive:

1. Repeat back key information patients told you. Yes, this may seem unnecessary because your brain is processing their input in a microsecond—but they will notice and appreciate it if you make this effort.
2. To drive the point home, plainly *state your intention* to repeat this information back. Saying, *"Let me summarize what I've heard you tell me"* is a simple, but highly effective, way to show patients that you listen well. And if it seems like a piece of information they've given is particularly important to them, be sure to acknowledge it.

EXPLAINING THINGS IN A WAY PATIENTS CAN UNDERSTAND

Medical jargon has a sneaky way of creeping into physicians' speech. It's difficult to eradicate entirely, but be on guard and do your best to avoid it when speaking to patients. For example:

- Borrow a tip from newspapers, which write to a middle-school reading level: Help ensure comprehension by using language at about an eighth-grade level.
- Ask, *"Was that clear?"* as your safety net for ensuring the patient fully understands.

- At the end of the visit, ask, *"Do you have any questions for me? I want to make sure you understand my thinking and agree with the plan going forward."*

SHOWING RESPECT FOR WHAT PATIENTS HAVE TO SAY

Most patients have stories to tell. It's their job, as your partner in the care process, to deliver relevant information so that you can provide the most fully informed clinical assessment of their situation.

To show respect for what patients tell you, take the following approach:

1. Acknowledge what you've heard by simply repeating back, in summary, what you've been told. To you, this may seem unnecessary because you know you've heard the information. But patients don't *know* you've heard it until you prove it by repeating it.

2. "Think out loud" to show patients how you're processing the information you've heard as you arrive at your clinical conclusions. Don't be afraid to gently say that some of the information they gave you probably doesn't affect your conclusions—but be sure to explain why. This discourse shows you heard what they said, even though it isn't related to what you think is the clinical issue.

If patients think something is important enough to mention, you'll be serving them best if you acknowledge it.

SPENDING ENOUGH TIME WITH PATIENTS

There is no specific, rule-of-thumb amount of time that is "enough." Your patients want you to spend whatever time is necessary to listen to their story, ask your questions, process the information (out loud), give recommendations for next steps, and ask if they have questions.

In other words, "enough time" is however long it takes for the patient to feel that the two of you have successfully accomplished your work together.

The biggest threat to "enough" is the *appearance* of being rushed. Again, perception is all-important. Giving your patients the sense that you are rushed introduces anxiety into the interaction: *"Is my doctor cutting corners? Will she miss or forget something because she's so busy?"*

Know Your Survey Questions

To do well in a game, you need to know how the score is kept.

In other words, you should know what questions your patients are being asked about you—what's on the survey. If you're not familiar with your organization's patient satisfaction survey, ask to take a look.

The questions on the survey weren't developed by chance. Survey vendors work with each client to obtain the data that will satisfy government reporting requirements and provide any additional information the client wants to collect about its patients' experience.

What follows is a sampling from the Hospital Consumer Assessment of Healthcare Providers and Systems (HCAHPS) survey, the CAHPS Clinician & Group (CG-CAHPS) doctor's office survey, a Press Ganey survey, and the Arbor Associates survey questions that correlate highly with overall patient satisfaction.

HCAHPS

Options for answering: Never, Sometimes, Usually, or Always.

- During this hospital stay, how often did doctors treat you with courtesy and respect?
- During this hospital stay, how often did doctors listen carefully to you?
- During this hospital stay, how often did doctors explain things in a way you could understand?

Source: HCAHPS (2014).

CG-CAHPS

Options for answering: Never, Sometimes, Usually, or Always.

- In the last 12 months, how often did this provider explain things in a way that was easy to understand?
- In the last 12 months, how often did this provider listen carefully to you?
- In the last 12 months, how often did this provider give you easy-to-understand information about these health questions or concerns?

(continued)

(continued from previous page)

- In the last 12 months, how often did this provider seem to know the important information about your medical history?
- In the last 12 months, how often did this provider show respect for what you had to say?
- In the last 12 months, how often did this provider spend enough time with you?
- Using any number from 0 to 10, where 0 is the worst provider possible and 10 is the best provider possible, what number would you use to rate this provider?

Source: AHRQ (2011).

Press Ganey

Options for answering. Rate the following areas on a numeric (Likert) scale:

- Friendliness/courtesy of the care provider
- Explanations the care provider gave you about your problem or condition
- Concern the care provider showed for your questions or worries
- Care provider's efforts to include you in decisions about your treatment
- Amount of time the care provider spent with you

Source: University of Utah Health Care (2016).

Arbor Associates

Options for answering. Rate the following areas on a numeric (Likert) scale:

- Inpatients:
  - Doctors did not listen carefully.
  - Not included in care, but wanted to be.
- Outpatients:
  - Doctors not friendly.
  - Doctors did not seem skilled.
  - Not included in discussing care, but wanted to be.
- Medical office:
  - Doctor never or only sometimes showed respect for what you had to say.
  - Doctor never or only sometimes knew about medical history.
  - Doctor never or only sometimes listened carefully.

(continued)

(continued from previous page)

    – Doctor never or only sometimes explained things in an easy-to-understand way.

    – Not included in discussing care, but wanted to be.

Source: D. Cohen, personal communication, March 10, 2014.

Your organization may use a survey with different questions. Know what they are! Your patients' satisfaction with you is being measured by their responses.

All doctors are incredibly busy people. You must walk the fine line between keeping things moving and not appearing overloaded. Your job is to protect your patients from the stress and anxiety inherent in the modern American medical system.

So, before you enter each room or patient cubicle, pause and put on your *calm* game face. Let the doctor patients see be in control of her day.

GIVING INFORMATION ABOUT TREATMENT

If you've demonstrated that you listened and then openly shared your thinking about your clinical conclusions, you've laid a great foundation for a positive interaction and relationship.

Most patient–physician exchanges are incomplete if they do not include discussion of treatment or next steps. Sometimes this discussion involves explaining and weighing options; sometimes the best course of action is clear. In either case, you should

- involve patients in making the decision, even if that means merely pausing and asking whether your recommendations make sense to them, and
- ask if patients have any questions about what lies ahead.

SHOWING CONCERN FOR PATIENTS' COMFORT

I once coached an emergency medicine doctor who personally offered each patient a warm blanket if he thought it might be needed. He enjoyed doing it, and the gesture made a huge, positive impression on his patients.

I'm not suggesting you go to that extreme. What we're really talking about here is being responsive to pain or any other discomfort. Helping patients ease their discomfort in the clinical environment may not score you extra points, but *not* responding to it will almost always cost you in their eyes.

Here is all you need to do: Ask about the patient's level of pain or discomfort and respond in some way. Sometimes your response might be prescribing pain medication, but often it can be as simple as bringing (or making sure another staff member brings) ibuprofen, another pillow, a throat lozenge, a blanket, a glass of water, some facial tissue, a packet of crackers, and so on. Most doctors do a good job at this. For those who make this effort, it's important to make absolutely certain the patient's request doesn't get overlooked during a handoff to a nurse or another member of the care team.

INCLUDING PATIENTS IN THEIR OWN CARE

It shouldn't come as a surprise that doctors who view their relationship with each patient as a partnership earn higher satisfaction ratings than those who perceive themselves as an authority figure. The partnership approach implies an open exchange of information and mutually agreed-upon decisions.

The following are some basic guidelines for establishing the physician–patient partnership dynamic:

- Give patients your undivided attention—really. Listen intently. Make their situation the only thing on your mind when you're with them.
- Interrupt only if you need to ask a question to probe deeper or understand clearly.
- When it comes time to ask your questions, help patients understand why you're seeking the information.
- Once you have all the data, keep talking—"think out loud"—to give patients a view into how your brain processes your findings from the physical exam, test results, and the history they have provided. This step increases your credibility and decreases their anxiety about what lies ahead. Then, when you ask, *"Does this sound like a reasonable way to proceed?"* you are more likely to get a "yes."

BEING FRIENDLY

I don't have a lot to say here that you don't already know. Being friendly won't earn you extra points (in fact, being extra-friendly can be creepy to some people). But *not* being friendly will cost you.

A few observations beyond the basics are as follows:

- A rushed doctor can seem cold and unfriendly.
- Small talk is good, but not necessary. Many doctors who aren't small-talkers do a great job conveying the message that they are very interested in their patients' well-being. Being an introvert does not mean you can't be highly engaged with your patient and his problem.
- If you're a natural with small talk, then by all means be friendly in your own way. Many patients enjoy amicable banter with their doctor if the situation isn't dire and the chatting doesn't detract from the business at hand.

INSPIRING FAITH IN THE PROVIDER'S CLINICAL ABILITIES

Although increased consumerism and the Internet are eroding blind trust in physicians' abilities, patients usually assume that you have good clinical skills. Reinforce their favorable assessment of you by keeping the following in mind:

- Patients may think you've forgotten an important point if you fail to acknowledge information they've given you. Remember to repeat it back, especially key points.
- Again, don't rush. It will make patients worry that you're cutting corners or that you might miss something.
- You take your abilities for granted, but your patients may not. To build trust, talk them through the process you've used to consider the information from the visit and how it supports the conclusions you're reaching.
- Language is powerful—even more so coming from a clinical expert such as yourself. Consider using these powerful phrases throughout an interaction to help patients appreciate your clinical abilities and collaborative style:
    - *"Here's what I've heard you say. . . ."*
    - *"Here's what the test results indicate. . . ."*
    - *"This is what I'm thinking. . . ."*
    - *"This is what I'm not thinking. . . ."* (patients value rule-outs).
    - *"Based on the information we've discussed, here are the next steps. . . ."*
    - *"Does this seem reasonable?"*

—   *"Based on all the information you've given me, the points that concern me most are . . ."* (for patients who have told you much more than you need to know).

In Part I, we've covered the specific behaviors physicians can adopt that maximize patient satisfaction and engagement (Chapter 1), and we've cross-walked those behaviors to correspond to the needs that patients have—as represented by patient satisfaction survey questions (Chapter 2).

In Part II, we address how you can tackle the deceptively difficult task of adopting these behaviors as every force in your daily life conspires against that effort.

REFERENCES

Agency for Healthcare Research and Quality (AHRQ). 2011. "CAHPS® Clinician & Group Surveys, 12-Month Survey 2.0, Adult." Updated September 1. www.cahps.ahrq.gov/surveys-guidance/cg/instructions/12monthsurvey.html.

Hospital Consumer Assessment of Healthcare Providers and Systems (HCAHPS). 2014. "HCAHPS Survey." www.hcahpsonline.org/surveyinstrument.aspx.

University of Utah Health Care. 2016. "About the Press Ganey Survey." Accessed May 6. http://healthcare.utah.edu/fad/pressganey.php.

Part II

HOW PHYSICIANS CAN MAKE AND SUSTAIN BEHAVIOR CHANGES

CHAPTER 3

The Science of Behavior Change

WHEN I WENT looking for resources to help physicians improve their interactions with patients, I found that most focus on the *whats*—what physicians should do (e.g., sit down, make eye contact, don't interrupt). While the whats are important, I've come to believe the more helpful question is *how*—

How *can doctors change ingrained behaviors successfully?*

Some of my clients have made changes quickly. So I've studied what they did and how they did it to develop a practical method for the how—a way to *execute and sustain* positive behavior changes that produce excellent interactions with patients—which I present in the next chapter.

Here, as an introduction to physician behavior change, I delve into the scientific basis of this method. It incorporates my experiences with successful doctors all over the country and draws significantly on wide-ranging research on change, improvement, and getting things done, including concepts from

- Prochaska and DiClemente's Stages of Change;
- Shewhart and Deming's Plan, Do, Study, Act (PDSA);
- Franklin Covey's *4 Disciplines of Execution*; and
- the Baldrige Performance Excellence Framework (Health Care).

STAGES OF CHANGE

The Stages of Change model was developed by James Prochaska and Carlos DiClemente (1983) from research into how people go about quitting smoking—some successfully, others not.

It identifies six stages in a successful change:

1. Pre-contemplation (including denial and unawareness)
2. Contemplation
3. Preparation for change
4. Action
5. Maintenance
6. Relapse

Helpful insights from this research include the following:

- Change is a process, and one must go through all the stages. If you don't start at the beginning, you'll almost certainly fail. (And doctors and other high-achieving people sometimes get ahead of themselves, don't they?) In other words, the act of *preparing to make* a change can prevent failure.
- Some people remain unaware of why making a change is important, even as many, or most, people around them fully understand that change is necessary.
- Personal change must come from internal motivation. It never comes from external influences.
- Help is needed to sustain a successful change.
- Relapse is to be expected. It does not mean failure, but it should be prepared for and can be successfully addressed.

PLAN, DO, STUDY, ACT

Walter Shewhart and his better-known protégé, W. Edwards Deming, introduced the concept of learning and improving not in a linear fashion but rather in cycles that build on knowledge gained from previous cycles. Known as PDSA, their methodology—which suggests to "design it, put it on the market, assess whether it works, re-design it, and start the process over again" (Moen and Norman 2014)—tends to be underappreciated in its applicability to a broad range of management (and personal) challenges. Many—maybe even most—problems can be attacked by trying a solution, assessing whether it leads to improvement, taking stock of what you've learned, making adjustments, and so on.

The key takeaways from PDSA are as follows:

- Progress is not linear but occurs in cycles. It comes from thoughtful trial and error and takes dedication, discipline, and patience. (A little stubbornness may also be helpful.) The extent to which you succeed is directly related to how long you're willing to keep trying.
- Because the process is cyclical, it never stops. The quest for improvement on a big goal is ongoing.
- Improvement can be best achieved systematically. It requires commitment to an important goal and to sustaining an ongoing process to achieve that goal.
- *Here's a big key:* Empiricism is important. Data, observations, and feedback are crucial for identifying needed changes and for building a knowledge base to guide and accelerate progress.

4 DISCIPLINES OF EXECUTION

The 4 Disciplines of Execution (McChesney, Covey, and Huling 2012) provides a framework for getting things done *even in the face of the "whirlwind"*—the day-to-day work of the organization that sucks time away from being able to focus on improving.

Key insights from the *4 Disciplines* concept include these:

- The daily challenges of getting the work done will always conspire to consume the time that could be devoted to figuring out how to do the work better. The urgent (which act on you) always wins out over the important (which you are trying to act on). And naturally, your job in caring for patients places urgency at the fore.
- When it comes to goals, less is more. The fewer goals you have, the more likely you are to achieve them. Having one to three goals is ideal. McChesney, Covey, and Huling (2012) remind us of this tenet using a classic line: "How do you eat an elephant? One bite at a time."
- *Here's another big key:* Act on lead measures, not lag measures. A lag measure, like your personal patient satisfaction percentile ranking, is useful as a long-term success indicator but cannot be acted on directly.

A lead measure, such as "I will always ask the patient if she has any more questions before I leave the room," can be acted on and improved—many times *today*.

- Create a compelling way to keep score. A good scorecard balances lag measures and lead measures. (See Appendix 5.4 in Chapter 5.)
- Improvement proceeds best through a regular schedule of accountability. For example, hold a weekly five-minute meeting with your colleagues to discuss progress on your few key goals, actions taken that week, and actions planned for next week. You can also hold a quarterly review of your patient satisfaction scores, preferably with your peers.

BALDRIGE PERFORMANCE EXCELLENCE FRAMEWORK

Ideas from the Health Care version of the Baldrige Excellence Framework (Baldrige Performance Excellence Program 2015) are also helpful. This framework is a series of questions used to develop high-performing organizations. My insights on the applicability of Baldrige to behavior change in physicians come from the framework itself; from Baldrige best-practice research by John Griffith, LFACHE, professor emeritus at the University of Michigan School of Public Health (Griffith and White 2005); and from my years of experience as a Baldrige examiner, Baldrige team leader, and former leader at a Baldrige National Quality Award–recipient organization.

(Perhaps your organization uses Baldrige principles to improve and measure its results. If not, the points I summarize here provide insight into ways the leaders of your group can support your efforts to improve. Sometimes all it takes is a suggestion from a single physician to get a performance improvement initiative launched in an organization.)

Key takeaways from the Baldrige framework are the following:

- Improvements are usually the result of a systematic and sustained effort (we've heard this before).
- Progress can be made and sustained, even after previous attempts have failed (sound familiar?).
- Periodically taking stock of strengths and opportunities for improvement is important—both to mark and celebrate progress and to recalibrate future priorities.
- Leadership plays an important role in setting and communicating priorities, ensuring that systematic approaches are followed, and

establishing a culture of accountability. (Note: Doctors *can* make improvements without leadership support if they have to; see Chapter 7.)

- Holding the workforce accountable (through a performance management system aligned with the few most important goals) can play a significant role in organizational performance. If your employer doesn't hold you accountable, you can benefit from holding yourself accountable.

- Thoughtfully recognizing and rewarding progress sustains and accelerates the journey. If your organization doesn't recognize and reward physicians with high or improving patient satisfaction scores, you should reward yourself to celebrate progress.

So now that we have a solid background in the science of making and sustaining changes, it's time to apply those concepts to the real world—*your* real world of too little time, heavy patient loads, and all the other challenges that abound in healthcare. Read on to Chapter 4.

REFERENCES

Baldrige Performance Excellence Program. 2015. "Baldrige Excellence Framework." Updated February 4. www.nist.gov/baldrige/publications/hc_criteria.cfm.

Griffith, J. R., and K. R. White. 2005. "The Revolution in Hospital Management." *Journal of Healthcare Management* 50 (3): 170–89.

McChesney, C., S. Covey, and J. Huling. 2012. *The 4 Disciplines of Execution: Achieving Your Wildly Important Goals.* New York: Free Press.

Moen, R., and C. Norman. 2014. "Evolution of the PDCA Cycle." Accessed January 24. http://pkpinc.com/files/NA01MoenNormanFullpaper.pdf.

Prochaska, J. O., and C. C. DiClemente. 1983. "Stages and Processes of Self-Change of Smoking: Toward an Integrative Model of Change." *Journal of Consulting and Clinical Psychology* 51 (3): 390–95.

CHAPTER 4

How to Make and Sustain Behavior Changes

WHEN I COACH physicians to address their challenges when interacting with patients, some make and sustain improvement. But others don't.

Why?

Because physicians are just people. And while most of us would say that becoming intentionally better at patient interactions is the right thing to do, it also means—for many physicians—changing ingrained behaviors. Just like quitting smoking or losing weight, any new behavior can be tough to adopt and stick to.

The most frequent request that I get from physician groups is "just tell us how to have great interactions with patients." And for years, I have given lots of talks about those key "make or break" elements of a typical patient interaction.

Unfortunately, those talks—alone—rarely lead to improvements. Even after individual coaching, this conversation happened too frequently:

Bo (to a client several months later): "Have you been able to make that key change we talked about?"

Physician client: "No, but I'll start working on it soon. Really, I promise." (Or, "Yes I have," as his nose begins to grow.)

Moving from a current state to any desired future state—even when you know *exactly* what that future state should look like—can be difficult. *And doctors face additional barriers:*

- You are incredibly busy. The time and energy that could be devoted to improvement are consumed by other urgent (some of them life-threatening) patient care issues.

- As high achievers, you often try to tackle too many changes at once and get overwhelmed.
- Because the behavior changes mentioned in Chapter 1 seem *simple,* you'll be tempted to make the mistake of discounting them as also being *easy.*
- You expect the rest of the world to be as efficient as you are, so you get impatient and frustrated with how long it takes for your hard work to show up in improved patient satisfaction scores, which are *lagging* indicators.

Changing behaviors does not come naturally to most of us. It takes awareness, introspection, motivation, and stick-to-it-iveness. And it helps if you can refer (and keep referring) to a simple model that has proved successful for others. So here it is.

MY PROVEN METHOD, IN A NUTSHELL

Stage 1: Become aware that a positive physician–patient interaction is very important and that *you* control whether this happens most of the time.

Stage 2: Thoughtfully take stock of how well you interact with patients, and prepare to undertake behavior changes to do it better.

Stage 3: Commit to one key change, and keep trying until you've mastered it.

Stage 4: Commit to making a second key change. Then continue the process as more changes are attempted, mastered, and sustained.

Stage 5: Don't rest on your laurels! Take stock of your progress on behaviors you've changed and identify future opportunities.

Elementary? Yes (and no).

I can hear you thinking, "Well, of course" to this process. But actually doing it will require more—keep reading.

As Woody Allen said in *Annie Hall,* "80 percent of success is showing up." The first challenge, and one of the biggest, is to truly engage on the topic of patient satisfaction.

I often encounter health system leaders who want to get right to the assessment and action stages when they still have physicians who are not yet engaged. It won't work. Organizations can help guide a doctor toward engagement, provide facilitation, and support her in her efforts—even require change as a condition of employment. But ultimately it's the doctor's choice. Will you engage and make changes, or not? Efforts brought on by external forces (the organization, your practice partners, and the like) will always fail if you haven't embraced the need to improve.

This is not getting ready to do the work. Getting ready *is part of* the work.

Stage 1: Building Awareness and Engagement, and Becoming Open to Change

The fact that you're reading this book indicates you are open to changing some behaviors. (If you need more convincing, skip ahead to Chapters 9 and 10 in Part IV.)

At this early awareness-building stage, ask yourself the following questions to get started:

- *How do I judge whether I'm doing a good job as a physician?* Be honest: Is "patient perception" on the list?
- *Am I "a natural" at engaging with patients?* Don't worry if you answer "no." In my experience, more than half of all doctors are not naturally at ease with patient interactions. If that's the case for you, ask yourself, What is my level of comfort in the typical patient interaction? Do I enjoy meeting patients for the first time? Do I dread it? Am I generally an introvert? An extrovert? Somewhere in between?
- *How long has it been since I've really paid attention to my patient satisfaction performance data?* What's my percentile ranking? Assuming the data are available to you, how often do you pay close attention? Frequently? Sometimes? Never?
- *Among members in my group, do formal or informal discussions about patient satisfaction take place?* Who usually brings it up? Do my colleagues have any discernible attitudes about patient satisfaction? Is anyone else interested in working on improving? If so, who?

Stage 2: Assessing, Learning, and Preparing to Change

This stage begins when you decide (and sincerely believe): "I'm totally aware of how important the physician–patient interaction is, and I understand that I can make some changes to do it better. *But now what do I do about it?*"

Remember, you're still in the thinking stages. (Note that a lot of this method is mental—luckily, doctors are good at that kind of thing!) Think about the following in preparation to make a change:

- What information do you need in order to learn *what* behaviors to change and *how* to change them? These new behaviors are not innate, instinctive, inborn—whatever word you want to use—for most of us. Performing them goes way beyond what we naturally do as "a good person." So at this point, you should acknowledge that it's time to get input from others.
  - Would a self-assessment help? Input from your colleagues or staff? Input from an internal or external coach?
- What do you see as potential barriers to successful change? Do any of these common obstacles apply to you?
  - Being too busy to focus on improving
  - Having a hard time hiding frustration from difficult patients or families
  - Language barriers
  - Difficulty sticking with an improvement journey
- What can you do to maintain focus and attention on improving when urgent matters distract you?
- Can you see a way your barriers can be overcome?

Stage 3: Making a *Singular* Change

Now that you are ready to attempt change, you must choose where to start.

Recall the insights I shared earlier from the book *The 4 Disciplines of Execution* (McChesney, Covey, and Huling 2012), the first of which is to have *only a few important goals*. Attempting to achieve more than a couple of objectives will cause you to lose focus, especially in the face of the whirlwind—the "real work" that must be done daily in your practice of medicine, the work that tries hard to eat up any time available to focus on improving.

As you decide which change to start with, consider information from your self-assessment, suggestions from others, and observations from patients (see Chapter 5) to develop a prioritized list of strengths and opportunities for improvement—a concept borrowed from the Baldrige Performance Excellence Framework (Baldrige Performance Excellence Program 2015).

Make—and Own—a Very Short List
Both of these aspects—making and owning—are necessary for success. First, you—not anyone else—must determine which improvement opportunities will be most significant for you.

When I shadow coach physicians, I can often identify the one or two opportunities that I think will make the biggest impact for them, and a lot of times we're on the same page. But when we're not, the doctor's preference generally trumps mine.

And second, if you don't "own" your list, it will be hard to make headway. Remember, Prochaska and DiClemente (1983) found that the motivation to change must come from within. You can always revise your list later.

As an example, let's say:

> You've decided to improve how you make a first impression on patients.

Try a Change and See How It Works

Here, you apply Shewhart and Deming's Plan-Do-Study-Act (PDSA) cycle of learning and improvement (introduced in Chapter 3) in a simple but focused way that has huge value. Choose a new behavior that may produce the change you'd like to see and test it on your next patient or your entire next day's schedule of patients.

> On Tuesday, you try the following process with each patient:
> 1. Knock on the door.
> 2. Say, with warmth and respect, "Good morning, Mrs. Green, I'm Dr. Smith. I'm your physician today. Is this a good time for me to come in and see you?"

Understand That Adjustment Is Expected

How'd it go?

Your first attempt probably won't go perfectly or smoothly. This may bug you. But recognize that the first time a new behavior is tried, it always feels awkward and won't go as well as you hoped. That's OK—PDSA is a cycle. You try something, you assess how it went, you try something different, you assess how well that went and what you learned, and so on.

> After a couple of awkward pauses in the hallway, you realize that you must step into the patient's view before you start speaking.

So tweak your approach.

Practice

Maybe different wording will make a new behavior more successful. Or using different body language. But most often, it's merely repeated practice that improves your comfort level with a new behavior. You must practice the new behavior until it is perfected *and becomes second nature.* Then keep practicing it, being careful to note with each interaction whether you performed it as desired.

> You're several weeks into practicing your new way to make a good first impression. It felt really weird at first, but as promised, through experimentation, repetition, and reflection, you've become comfortable using different wording that doesn't sound robotic. It now feels natural, and you decide to try adding a new line when appropriate, such as, *"May I pull up a chair so we can talk more comfortably?"*
>
> After several more weeks of experimenting, you decide that you are very much at ease with your new skills at making a warm first impression. In fact, you suddenly realize you're doing it without thinking about it!

It's time to move on to your next opportunity for improvement.

How Long Will It Take?

Work on one key priority for two weeks to a month. Depending on the individual physician, the time it takes to perfect a new behavior can be longer or shorter.

And remember, it's usually not difficult to do something differently. What's hard is doing something differently *every time* without thinking about it. Only time and practice will ingrain a behavior.

A standard analogy is learning a new language and finally having a dream in that language for the first time. That's the level of familiarity one needs to reach before moving on to the next opportunity. And this always takes a while.

The time frame also depends on the nature of the behavior that's being changed. Adjusting your approach to make a great first impression can be worked on with each new patient. But avoiding arguments with difficult patients will take longer because those situations happen less frequently.

What About Tackling a Broader Change?

Physicians who have significant work to do on their interactions with patients can sometimes benefit from making broader, more fundamental changes first. Here's an example:

> Before visiting every patient, I will pause and imagine that I am walking on stage to perform before 5,000 people, including the toughest critic from the *New York Times*. My goal is for the review in tomorrow's paper to be glowing.

I've seen that a broad focus on overall awareness really helps doctors who chronically interact poorly with patients. They need to take a preliminary step to consciously bring the issue of patient engagement front and center just prior to each encounter. Once that occurs consistently, they begin to make more specific changes.

Of course, a broad change doesn't work for everybody. Some doctors are so uncomfortable with the thought of doing *anything* differently that they may have to initially focus on the very simplest and most specific change, perhaps as basic as:

> I will look the patient in the eye and shake his hand when introducing myself.

On the flip side, doctors who generally perform well with patients may benefit only from narrow, specific change opportunities because they already understand the big picture.

The beauty of applying PDSA is that it won't let you make a long-term mistake—you try something for a while, then assess whether it's making a difference. Then you decide what to do next based on what you've learned.

Stage 4: Choosing the Next Change

Once you have implemented a new behavior, practiced it, and feel it has become second nature to your routine, it's time to choose the next change to make.

This process may be as simple as looking back at the prioritized list of opportunities you developed in Stage 3. If you tried a broad approach for your first change (e.g., *"I will pause before each patient interaction and remember that connecting with this patient will be important to his health outcome"*), you may be ready to try a more targeted second change:

> I will not interrupt patients, even a little, until they have been talking for at least 90 seconds (unless it's absolutely necessary or they're getting totally off topic; then I'll redirect them as gently as I can).

Once you've chosen your second change opportunity, you can begin experimenting by practicing it with patients until you command it. Then you choose your next priority, and the cycle continues.

This method takes tremendous discipline. And you—like the rest of us—will never be "done" improving. But the process is incredibly rewarding personally, professionally, perhaps financially—you name it. In my experience, doctors are energized by their first success and are eager to continue. It's like losing weight. The first five pounds are the hardest. Unlike losing weight, where the pounds can come back on, it's harder to revert to old habits once you've ingrained a new behavior. But it can happen, so we address that next.

Stage 5: Sustaining Each Change and Your Broader Journey

Once you've successfully changed a behavior or two, it's important not to take your victories for granted or lose focus on your personal improvement journey. Why stop improving when you have more opportunities ahead?

A number of doctors I've worked with have achieved 99th percentile patient satisfaction scores. The reason they score so high and sustain those high scores is that they never stop focusing on improving patient satisfaction.

Once a physician achieves a high-performing state, she has to use less energy to sustain it. To solidify your behavior changes, consider taking the following steps (and find more resources for sustaining improvement in Part III):

- Keep a weekly journal or log. This can be shared if you're working with a buddy or in a group (see Chapter 5). But it can also be helpful just for yourself—to keep track of progress and plans for future actions. The tool used for your journal need not be cumbersome or complex—jot a few notes on a sheet of paper, sticky note, smartphone, or tablet in less than a minute once a week. The key is to stick with the process and continually review your success.

- Trade weekly e-mails with an appointed coach. The coach may be a colleague who's a superstar at patient interaction, in a sort of buddy system. Or he may be another leader in the organization or an external person skilled at coaching on the subject. This practice will hardwire a weekly reflection into your schedule, provide an opportunity to share progress and barriers, and inject both support and recommendations on how best to proceed through difficult periods when it seems like little progress is being made. A weekly e-mail can take less than five minutes, and being accountable to another person in this reciprocal way can keep you focused.

- Periodically review new, relevant data, such as patient complaints or compliments received through e-mail, verbatim responses to the patient satisfaction survey, or unsolicited notes of appreciation or complaint.

Asking that this kind of feedback be included in monthly or quarterly staff meetings is one way to make sure you have access to it on a regular basis.

- Review your individual patient satisfaction scores and percentile ranking whenever the sample size yields meaningful data. This metric is the ultimate lagging indicator and the periodic "moment of truth." If you're not seeing your numeric patient satisfaction score, you should work with your leader to get it (more on this topic in Chapter 6).

In Part II, we've covered the important basics of how to go about making and sustaining behavior changes. Part III, "Resources for the Improvement Journey," provides additional insights and practical tools to support your progress.

REFERENCES

Baldrige Performance Excellence Program. 2015. *2015–2016 Baldrige Excellence Framework: A Systems Approach to Improving Your Organization's Performance (Health Care)*. Gaithersburg, MD: US Department of Commerce, National Institute of Standards and Technology.

McChesney, C., S. Covey, and J. Huling. 2012. *The 4 Disciplines of Execution: Achieving Your Wildly Important Goals*. New York: Free Press.

Prochaska, J. O., and C. C. DiClemente. 1983. "Stages and Processes of Self-Change of Smoking: Toward an Integrative Model of Change." *Journal of Consulting and Clinical Psychology* 51 (3): 390–95.

Part III

RESOURCES FOR THE IMPROVEMENT JOURNEY

CHAPTER 5

Tools for First Steps

In Chapter 4, we covered the logic behind how to make changes in your routine to have better interactions with patients. In this chapter, we discuss specific tools to help you begin and sustain your journey.

Whether you have help from your practice or health system (I outline how they can help you in the next chapter) or are embarking on the improvement journey on your own (take heart, and see Chapter 7), you can benefit from the practical tools in this chapter:

1. A self-assessment specially designed to help you make the biggest impact
2. A "where to start" worksheet
3. A tool for collecting the thoughts of others
4. A scorecard and personal action plan to help you maintain focus and track your progress over the long term

You can start with a simple awareness "cheat sheet"—Exhibit 1.1 in Chapter 1. It groups dozens of specific, high-impact change opportunities by the chronology of a typical patient visit. I suggest photocopying it and posting it in a place where you'll see it regularly.

SELF-ASSESSMENT

Doctors preparing to make behavior changes should complete a self-assessment, such as the tool provided in Appendix 5.1. This exercise will help prepare you for the improvement journey ahead and identify behavior changes that will make the biggest impact. Topics addressed can include the following:

- Describing your personal style of interacting with patients
- Identifying your greatest strengths when interacting with patients
- Identifying one or two specific behaviors you could change to make the most positive impact on your patients' impressions of you
- Identifying your biggest concerns about the barriers that might keep you from providing a better interaction with your patients
- Thinking about how your patients might be rating your interactions with them
- Reviewing your most recent personal patient satisfaction survey scores and verbatim comments from patients
- Reviewing formal thank-you notes or complaints from patients

Take your time completing this self-assessment, be honest with yourself, and see it as an investment in your professional development.

"WHERE TO START" WORKSHEET

No one can remember, let alone improve, every component of a typical patient interaction. To keep those one to three most significant potential changes at the top of your mind, consider rank-ordering your opportunities. The "where to start" worksheet in Appendix 5.2 lists the components of a typical patient interaction, which correspond to the items in our nuts-and-bolts framework for engaging patients (Exhibit 1.1).

You can think of the self-assessment and the "where to start" worksheet as opposite sides of the same coin. The former asks you to think about your opportunities without prompts; the latter offers prompts. Try doing both, starting with the unprompted self-assessment, and see what insights they lead you to.

WAYS TO COLLECT THE OPINIONS OF OTHERS

The self-assessment is most helpful when you review it in tandem with others' assessments of you. Objective observers such as the following can provide valuable information:

- *A professional coach* (full disclosure: I am one). It's the coach's job to identify strengths and challenges and communicate them supportively as he shadows and observes a physician.

Specifically, a shadow coach observes doctor–patient interactions, taking note of how the patient is reacting, how the coach would react if he were the patient, and how the coach might handle the situation if he were the doctor. The coach provides individualized feedback on observed strengths and recommends opportunities for improvement.

- *An internal coach.* Some organizations have developed internal coaches for these types of observations—and have achieved rewarding results. Chapter 8 of my companion book (Snyder 2016) gives an in-depth discussion on how to develop this capacity within an organization.

- *Staff members and peer colleagues.* You may seek input from the nurse you work closest with, medical assistants, or other caregivers who orbit around you and observe your interactions with patients. When approaching observers among staff, (1) let them know why you are interested in getting feedback and why honesty is important to the helpfulness of the feedback, and (2) follow up with a paper questionnaire that your staff observers can complete without identifying themselves—if that makes them more comfortable giving frank feedback.

  The same approach can be used to engage physician partners in a group. Depending on the culture in your practice, collecting your part- ners' input can be accomplished through frank, reciprocal discussions, prefaced with a statement such as, *"If you tell me honestly how you think I'm doing with patients, I'll do the same for you."* You could also solicit written feedback that can be signed or unsigned. Appendix 5.3 provides sample staff and peer questionnaires.

- *And of course, patients.* The most meaningful observations here are mined via the "free-text" feedback from patient satisfaction surveys and unsolicited notes of appreciation or complaint.

Remember, the numeric scores tabulated at the end of a reporting period (often when the sample size becomes large enough to draw a meaningful conclusion) are *lagging* indicators. They are very important but can't be influenced immediately.

A more directly helpful kind of patient feedback are the verbatim survey com- ments (*leading* indicators that can be acted on)—sometimes reported in batches, but more helpfully reported in real-time feedback that can be used for more imme- diate service recovery. For example, a patient's report that *"Dr. Smith basically just walked out of the room when I clearly had unanswered questions"* is excellent feed- back for Dr. Smith to consider as he prioritizes his personal plan of action.

And sometimes patients give feedback even more directly. Occasionally they are brave enough to confront their doctor during or immediately after the visit, but more commonly they speak to a nurse or another staff member. Sometimes a complaint is relayed from a patient to a family member who contacts another person on the care team or the hospital's patient relations department.

Regardless of the source and type of feedback, your organization should be providing it to you. If you're not getting it, ask for it.

SCORECARD AND PERSONAL ACTION PLAN

The final tool we discuss in this chapter is a combination scorecard and action plan to help you maintain focus and track your progress over the longer term. As you review the sample in Appendix 5.4, note that this scorecard and plan can take any number of forms. I encourage you to develop whatever format works for you. It might be as simple as a single-page, handwritten document. However, I do suggest that you include the following core elements:

- A history of your individual patient satisfaction scores, listed as a percentile (reflecting how you rank against similar physicians in your specialty)
- Your group's overall patient satisfaction score
- The scores of all the other doctors in the group
- Recent unsolicited patient complaints or compliments with specific issues noted
- Specific, verbatim patient comments from satisfaction surveys
- A summary of your strengths (that you compile from assessments)
- A prioritized list of opportunities for improvement (OFIs) (also derived from the assessments)
- Which OFI you are working on now
- Which OFIs you have successfully converted to strengths or improved with past effort

Taking the time to develop and update such materials is important for several good reasons:

1. It is tremendously satisfying to track changes that you've made and sustained over a long-term horizon.
2. A scorecard/action plan keeps the patient satisfaction improvement process active. It establishes and maintains focus.

3.   The tool also balances short-term actions taken (fed by leading indicators) with movement in patient satisfaction scores (lagging indicator). If the needle isn't yet moving on the survey results, you can find some satisfaction in your progress with addressing opportunities as you interact with patients day to day.

4.   The scorecard also helps you sustain changes once they've been made. If you get so far as to work through all your OFIs, you can recalibrate—recycle former challenges already addressed back onto your scorecard to make sure they are revisited and maintained.

This chapter presents some tools and insights that you can use to assess which behavior changes to attempt and how to take stock of your efforts as you continue your journey. I hope your organization will be able to help you, at least to some degree. That is the topic of Chapter 6.

REFERENCE

Snyder, B. 2016. *The Best Patient Experience: Helping Physicians Improve Care, Satisfaction, and Scores*. Chicago: Health Administration Press.

Appendix 5.1 Sample Self-Assessment for Physicians

What to do with your completed assessment can vary greatly depending on your personal needs and those of your organization. Options:

- Save it. Refer to it later to privately assess progress.
- Share it with your peers at an upcoming staff meeting.
- Share it with your leader in a one-on-one discussion.
- Combine the results with input from your peers, coach, survey data, and so on to create a complete picture of your strengths and opportunities for improvement.

(continued)

Self-Assessment of Your Interactions with Patients

Instructions: This self-assessment relates to your interactions with your patients and your patients' subsequent impressions of you. Take enough time to answer these questions thoughtfully, but consider that your first impressions are often the most accurate.

Which description best fits you?

_____ How my patients think about me is very important to me. And I seem to be good at having positive interactions with them. I don't have to think about it—I'm a natural.

_____ How my patients think about me is very important to me. And I have put time, thought, and energy into having positive interactions with them.

_____ I don't think about my interactions with patients much, but I don't feel my interactions are perceived poorly. My main goal is to provide good clinical care.

_____ No one's ever thought of me as much of a "people person." My priority is to see a heavy case load each day and provide good clinical care.

If none of these descriptions hits the mark, jot down a sentence that more accurately describes your personal style in interacting with patients and where that fits in your professional priorities:

When it comes to interacting with patients, what are your greatest strengths? Limit your answers to a few of the biggest:

What one specific behavior could you change—either start doing or stop doing—to most positively influence your patients' impressions of you?

(continued)

When answering the previous question, did you think of additional behaviors that you could change to make an impact? List two or three of them here:

What do you see as the most significant barriers that might keep you from initiating and sustaining better interaction with your patients?

How do you think your patients rate your interactions with them?

_____ Much higher than with most other providers in your specialty

_____ Somewhat higher than with most other providers in your specialty

_____ About the same as with most other providers in your specialty

_____ Somewhat lower than with most other providers in your specialty

_____ Much lower than with most other providers in your specialty

If you have access to patient satisfaction survey data, what were your impressions of your most recent personal scores? What did you take away from those data?

How often do you

- receive formal (written/e-mailed) thank-yous from satisfied patients? Are there any themes?

- receive informal (verbal) thank-yous from satisfied patients? Any themes?

- receive formal (written or e-mailed) complaints from dissatisfied patients? Any themes?

Appendix 5.2 Worksheet: Where to Start—Identifying Your Single, Most Potentially Significant Behavior Change

Instructions: Pick three behavior changes to consider, and rank-order them, with 1 being the single most significant change you can make. That's the change—the only change—to start working on first. (If your specialty involves other key behaviors not listed here, by all means, write them in.)

Self-awareness

Awareness of
    circumstances

Awareness of patients'
    unique needs

Your greeting

Giving ways to remember
    your name

Asking permission using
    "May I?" and "Does that
    seem reasonable?"

Your body language and
    positioning

Using an open-ended first
    question

Having a communications
    plan

Sharing your clinical
    reasoning

Acknowledging discomfort

Showing respect when
    touching the patient

Using simpler language

Compensating for your
    accent

Interrupting gently

Repeating back

Disagreeing thoughtfully

Avoiding terms of
    endearment

Monitoring style and tone

Inserting speed bumps into
    your routine

Acknowledging wait times

Transitioning care to
    another provider with
    clarity

Clearly signaling the end of
    the interaction

Getting points for ensuring
    privacy

Using a closing summary

Describing next steps

Giving clear instructions

Offering re-clothing
    instructions

Making referrals

Posing a final question:
    "Any questions or
    concerns?"

Saying a warm good-bye

Other: _____

Other: _____

Note:

- This exercise will be easier if you've already invested time in a self-assessment (Appendix 5.1) or in gathering input from staff or peers (Appendix 5.3).

- It will be helpful to record your most important behavior change on your phone, your tablet, or even a sticky note—placed where you'll see it often.

- Keep a copy of this appendix in a location you'll remember—for reference later.

Appendix 5.3 Staff and Peer Questionnaires

Request for Feedback on My Interactions with Patients

To: My Valued Team Member   From: _____

Would you please help me by providing some feedback? I would like to improve how I interact with patients to help our team earn higher satisfaction scores. I'm interested in your candid assessment of my strengths and weaknesses in this area.

Note: Your feedback can be anonymous, if desired. *Please put your completed questionnaire in an envelope and place it in my mailbox.*

1. When it comes to interacting with patients, what are my one or two greatest strengths?

2. What *one* specific behavior could I change to most positively affect my patients' impressions of me? (This is something I could start doing, stop doing, or do more consistently to make the biggest impact.)

3. Once I successfully address this one issue, what are one to three other behaviors I could change to improve my patients' impressions of me?

Going forward, I ask that you help me by:

- Occasionally asking me what I'm currently focused on to serve patients better. I intend to always be working on something important. Your reminders will help me stay focused.
- Letting me know whenever you feel I could have handled a situation with a patient better, or when you think I handled a situation exceptionally well.
- Letting me know if a patient compliments or critiques my behavior.

You may include your name if you would like, but this is certainly not required: _____

Thank you! I appreciate your candid feedback and ongoing support.

Request for Feedback on My Interactions with Patients

To: My Valued Colleague   From: _____

Would you please help me by providing some feedback? I would like to improve how I interact with patients to help our team earn higher satisfaction scores. I'm interested in your candid assessment of my strengths and weaknesses in this area.

Note: Your feedback can be anonymous, if desired. *Please put your completed questionnaire in an envelope and place it in my mailbox.*

1. When it comes to interacting with patients, what are my one or two greatest strengths?

2. What *one* specific behavior could I change to most positively affect my patients' impressions of me? (This is something I could start doing, stop doing, or do more consistently to make the biggest impact.)

3. Once I successfully address this one issue, what are one to three other behaviors I could change to improve my patients' impressions of me?

You may include your name if you would like, but this is certainly not required: _____

Thank you! I truly appreciate your candid feedback and ongoing support.

Appendix 5.4 Sample Patient Satisfaction Scorecard and Action Plan

For: _____ Ben Smith _____

Time Period	My Percentile Score	Group's Percentile Score	My Ranking in the Group
4th quarter	21st	59th	7 of 8
1st quarter	38th	65th	6 of 8
2nd quarter	70th	68th	4 of 8
			___ of ___
			___ of ___
			___ of ___

Strengths

I don't use medical jargon.

I make a good first impression. I'm comfortable introducing myself and making eye contact with patients.

I make a good last impression. I always leave by wishing them a good day or a "hope you feel better soon."

Opportunities for Improvement

I can be a little blunt with patients who disagree with my clinical judgment.

I interrupt patients to ask them questions and keep things moving.

I typically don't ask if they have questions. If they have a question, they can ask. I don't want to give them permission to keep me in the room longer than necessary.

(continued)

(continued from previous page)

Sample Monthly Journal

Time Period	Actions and Observations
January	Just got our personal scores for the 1st time. Mine stink. I've never really thought much about the importance of my interactions with patients before. I just assumed I was doing OK. This is a wakeup call. I'm going to focus on the importance of a good interaction every time. Also being patient with rambling patients.
February	I'm letting patients talk for at least a minute before I interrupt. It's really hard when they're just rambling. Sometimes I just want to die!!!!! I got 2 patient complaints. One was from a patient with a crazy family. Marcus Welby couldn't have satisfied them. The other one was legit, in hindsight. We had differing opinions. My logic was on solid ground, but I think I came off like a jerk. I could have handled that better.
March	When they ramble, I play a game to see how I can diplomatically get them to keep moving. I'm getting better at this. I still try to remind myself before I go into the room that I haven't done a good job unless the patient is very satisfied with the way I treat them.
April	Hey, my score improved to 38th percentile. I'm ahead of Sarah now. We started to buddy in a friendly competition to see who could improve the most. We e-mail each other every week with what we're focusing on. I'm working on asking to make sure the patient doesn't have any questions.
May	Still working on asking for questions. I got another complaint about arguing with a patient. The thing about this one was I knew I wasn't being at my best right after I argued with them. But I was tired and I moved on without apologizing. At least I now know when I'm entering the DANGER ZONE!!
June	Still asking for questions. Now also working on summarizing the conversation at the end. Funny thing. When I do that there seem to be fewer questions.

(continued)

(continued from previous page)

July	Scores are way up!!! 70th percentile!! I passed RJ and Philip. My scores are a little bit better than the group average! Still working on summarizing, asking for questions, and making sure I show the patient how I'm processing all the information to arrive at the best recommendation for what should happen next. I avoided a confrontation with one family who was looking for a fight!

Patient Satisfaction Scorecard and Action Plan

For: _____

Time Period	My Percentile Score	Group's Percentile Score	My Ranking in the Group
			_____ of _____
			_____ of _____
			_____ of _____
			_____ of _____
			_____ of _____
			_____ of _____
			_____ of _____
			_____ of _____
			_____ of _____
			_____ of _____
			_____ of _____
			_____ of _____

Strengths

Opportunities for Improvement

Monthly Journal

Time Period	Actions and Observations

Monthly Journal

Time Period	Actions and Observations

CHAPTER 6

16 Ways Your Organization Can Help You Improve

THE BEST HEALTHCARE organizations not only require their physicians to have positive interactions with patients, but they also intentionally and systematically support their doctors' efforts to do so. Everyone in the organization is held accountable for providing a positive experience for the patient. With organizational support, progress is faster, relapses are less likely, and it's also less likely that doctors' efforts are abandoned in the face of the daily whirlwind.

If you belong to such an organization, congratulations! If you don't, read on. You may be able to introduce these ideas to the leaders in your practice or health system.

"Do as I Say, Not as I Do": A Formula for Physician Disgruntlement

Physicians become particularly frustrated when leaders (whether of hospitals or large group practices) nag them about their low patient satisfaction scores without offering support, or the leaders fail to hold similarly accountable all the staff who could make a positive contribution to the patient experience.

If you find yourself in this situation, you can diplomatically and firmly point out to the leaders just how ineffective this approach is (perhaps referring them to the first book in this series, which I refer to as "the leader book" [Snyder 2016]). Otherwise, your best option may be to ignore them and do the best you can or find a practice with more enlightened leadership.

A Forward-Thinking Way That One Organization Is Helping Its Doctors

Stanford Health Care, the academic health system affiliated with Stanford University, has used an array of integrated approaches to improve its physicians' patient satisfaction scores. According to Amir Dan Rubin, former president and CEO, Stanford Health Care has helped doctors accomplish this goal by following these practices (personal communication, November 5, 2014):

- Making the right hire
- Setting expectations during the on-boarding process
- Providing coaching for doctors who need further support
- Tracking and reporting results
- Offering formal and informal rewards and recognition
- Tying physician compensation to results

But Stanford Health Care is also borrowing a page from the review website Yelp. The organization plans to place all patient satisfaction survey comments online, where anyone can search them by physician, as well as verbatim (other than minor edits for clarity and appropriateness).

According to Rubin,

> Organizations like Healthgrades are inviting patients to comment on their doctors in public forums for everyone to review. *This is going to happen whether we want it to or not.* If we do it ourselves, patients and prospective patients will turn to us as the trusted resource for information. And we want them to do that.
>
> We have the added benefit of having the data come from a source we and our doctors trust and are familiar with. We have high expectations and an improvement mentality, so why wouldn't we be willing to make this data accessible? And knowing that the data will be public is a strong motivator to act in a way that will make [the organization] look good.

This method *does* help doctors. It creates unassailable transparency and a very strong incentive for *every* physician to perform highly in this area— great news to the doctors who care about the patient experience and are

(continued)

(continued from previous page)

working to improve. There's no way their colleagues who don't care can free-ride on their hard work.

Rubin says Stanford Health Care's approaches have paid off: Scores have risen from the 45th to the 95th percentile for inpatients, from the 10th to the 90th percentile in its cancer centers, and from the 15th to the 70th percentile in its outpatient clinics and medical group.

Note: Publishing comments online for the public to view was a natural extension of the system Stanford Health Care already had in place to help its physicians interact better with patients: They had all been working at this for a while. If your organization is at square one, it is not a good idea to put physician-specific comments online as a first step!

Many of the 16 approaches discussed here are group activities, but some can be used by an individual doctor who wants to make progress on her own, even if her group or employer is not providing help (more on these in Chapter 7). Although many of these approaches cost little to implement, most require the commitment, discipline, and sweat of the organization *as well as* of the individual.

That said, the following ways that forward-thinking organizations support their physicians' efforts to improve the patient experience, when adopted with an ownership mentality by both leadership and physicians, greatly improve the odds that improvement is made and sustained.

OVERARCHING MANAGEMENT PHILOSOPHIES

1. *The leaders establish the initiative with a consistent approach and message that they believe in.* A big job of leaders is to set direction. They talk about vision and priorities, and they are serious about the experiences that patients have. They insist that *everybody* is responsible for making that experience positive, both at the level of personal behavior and at an organizational level (e.g., addressing operational issues, such as shortening long wait times).

2. *The leaders do the work of improving.* Effective leaders roll up their sleeves and participate in making changes. They carve out time for discussions about which improvements will have the biggest impact. They ask doctors for input, especially on what the organization can do to help them have better interactions with their patients—decision making is inclusive.

   Once identified, improvement initiatives are rolled out with a game plan, and not all at once. Decisions are supported with follow-through to ensure proper execution and thoughtful assessment of whether further changes need to be made to enhance the improvement effort.

3. *The leaders embrace accountability.* In the best organizations, employees who don't take the patient experience seriously suffer consequences. Those who just give it lip service are eventually exposed. Knowing that they are accountable motivates people to engage and make the effort, it helps those who are unengaged to volunteer to work elsewhere, and it creates a culture that attracts those who want to be accountable for serving patients exceptionally well. (In the "Team Management" section of this chapter, we discuss rewards, recognition, and dealing with low performers.)

   Baldrige Award–recipient organizations report success when they have held *each employee* accountable for one or two specific behaviors that improve interactions with patients. Furthermore, the best healthcare organizations hold *leaders* accountable for patient satisfaction scores. Practice administrators are accountable, as are the hospital system leaders who manage those administrators. The system CEO should have concrete, measurable reasons to care about patient satisfaction throughout the organization. Everyone should have skin in the game.

   As a doctor on the front line, you have the powerful advantage of being able to control your personal scores. Those above you in the chain of command don't have that ability. So leading healthcare organizations *embed patient satisfaction into their employed providers' accountability standards* through the organization's performance management system, if applicable, or through the credentialing process. This step ensures that doctors receive a formal review of how well they are handling interactions with patients at least once each year.

PATIENT SURVEYS AND DATA

4. *Surveys are fielded with a large enough sample size to be helpful.* Some organizations invest in a patient satisfaction survey only to meet the minimum requirements of the Centers for Medicare & Medicaid Services. Healthcare organizations should invest not only in a quality survey but also in collecting enough completed surveys to yield *statistically significant* data that can be reviewed at a *doctor-specific level* several times each year. Survey results with a large enough sample size can provide that.

   If you're not getting this depth of feedback, approach your organization's leaders to start providing it. For all the reasons presented earlier in the book, you need to know how you're doing and the ultimate impact of any behavior changes you've made.

5. *Surveys give clean data for each doctor.* Often, data on patient satisfaction for inpatients are sorted by discharge physician. But what if a hospitalist discharges a patient whom he saw only once—on the day of discharge—and the patient had been served by two other hospitalists during his seven-day stay? In this case, the discharge doctor "gets credit" for the care provided by his colleagues over the days prior to discharge. This system may unfairly penalize or boost the scores attributed to the discharging doctor.

    Ask your organization to work with its survey vendor to provide "cleaner" data for each doctor. Although it may be nearly impossible to provide perfectly clean data for inpatient satisfaction because inpatients are often seen by many doctors, for an additional expense, the vendor *can* sort the data so that the majority of a doctor's score is based on care he (as opposed to other physicians) has provided.

    The bottom line is, while this level of data cleaning may be more expensive, the data lack credibility without it.

6. *Verbatim patient feedback, complaints, and compliments are actively used.* Most surveys give patients an opportunity to provide direct feedback through an open-ended comment section. Leading organizations quickly report these comments to the doctor so that she can benefit from the feedback. I recommend also including any compliments or complaints made to the hospital's patient relations department (or the similar department in your organization). Finally, as discussed further in the next paragraph, verbatim comments should be compiled in such a way that trends can be identified.

ADMINISTRATIVE SUPPORT

7. *Administrative support is provided to pull together the data and information*—numeric survey data, verbatim comments from the surveys, and unsolicited compliments and complaints—that each doctor needs to review his performance and monitor improvement. Some organizations have staff support to do this; others include this function in the standard work of the leader of each department (Barnas 2011).

    Regardless of the role structure, the best organizations have the following in place:

    • A person in charge of making the raw survey data understandable
    • A template to present the information in a standard format

- A schedule for presenting the patient feedback to the doctors regularly
- Agreed-upon ways in which the feedback will be followed up on (such as the scorecard and personal action plan shown in Appendix 5.4).

MAINTAINING A SCHEDULE OF ACCOUNTABILITY, OFTEN AS A GROUP

8. *Leading organizations use ongoing, frequent group check-ins* to help doctors maintain focus on the behavior changes they're addressing. One approach is to convene daily or weekly huddles to quickly recap progress. In this quick roundtable, physicians share their progress on individual changes—each talking for no more than 15 seconds. Think of this as essentially a verbal version of the "confessionals" process used so successfully by First Physician Corporation (FPC; see the case study in Chapter 8). Group check-ins can also be done via e-mail if timing and location don't allow for face-to-face gatherings.

9. *Patient satisfaction scores are reviewed with doctors on a regular basis.* Ideally, this includes results for each physician plus aggregate data for the group as a whole. If your organization does not have a helpful format for conveying the results, share the sample PowerPoint images in Appendix 6.1, at the end of this chapter, with your administrative leaders. It shows how to succinctly present the data in two ways: in a time series to demonstrate improvement and in comparison form to measure against peers or benchmarks.

10. *Other progress-sharing mechanisms are created and supported.* Some organizations ask everyone in the group to report the personal improvement they're working on to the administrator every few months. FPC summarized its physicians' confessionals into a report that was e-mailed to everyone in the group. Other groups publish updates in a newsletter.

    Some organizations share survey results at monthly or quarterly meetings, where each member of the group makes a brief report on the behavior change he or she is working on and what progress has been made. Appendix 6.1 includes a slide that can be used to guide the discussion.

TOOLS AND EDUCATION

11. *Effective self-help tools are made available for physicians.* These resources include the templates found in the Chapter 5 appendixes (self-assessment,

relationship-building behaviors inventory, staff and peer feedback questionnaires, and personal scorecard/action plan). In addition, leaders or support staff are available to help doctors get the most value from each tool.

In recognition that helping you improve has to consist of more than just saying, "Let's try to find a conference on the patient experience; I've got some money budgeted for that," high-performing organizations tend to also provide other substantive, vetted resources for learning and development. These resources can include supplying copies of this book, providing time with a mentor or coach, setting up roundtables or workshops with an expert, helping you complete a self-assessment, or compiling your staff or peer assessments.

COACHING

12. *One or more types of coaching are made available.* A shadow coach, for example, is an outside expert or a specially trained internal coach who spends time observing the doctor as she works with patients and then gives feedback and advice.

In another form of coaching, a skilled colleague could be appointed as a mentor to a less-skilled doctor, who follows along as the role model sees patients. In this form, mentor and mentee typically touch base on an ongoing basis to share information and chart progress.

Finally, the coaching relationship can be as simple as the doctor trading regular e-mails with a colleague who's a superstar at patient interaction in a sort of buddy system, with another leader in the organization, or with an external person skilled at coaching on this subject. Typically taking less than five minutes a week, this practice hardwires into your busy schedule a periodic (perhaps weekly) reflection, giving you the chance to share progress or challenges. It supports your efforts to keep going through difficult periods when it seems like little progress is being made.

TEAM MANAGEMENT

13. *Organizations provide formal rewards and recognition—both for individuals and for whole groups.* A rewards-and-recognition program encourages doctors to continue their hard work. Because praise from a colleague is one of the most powerful tools to reinforce behavior, physicians are given ample opportunities to relate their progress and milestones achieved and

to receive acknowledgment from colleagues and staff. Each physician learns from the others, and the stragglers are more likely to take the first steps past awareness to assessing, learning, preparing to change, and ultimately trying to change.

Leading organizations make a big deal out of progress in a variety of ways—from awarding pizza parties and movie tickets to using individual or group performance to determine how vacation time is allotted or incentive bonuses are paid.

14. *Team members are screened effectively.* Prospective physicians are evaluated for whether they will be good at interacting with patients, and high-performing organizations don't hire candidates who clearly have problems in this area. Their leaders would rather leave a position open or fill it with a *locum tenens* than take someone they suspect will deliver lower-than-tolerable patient satisfaction scores and higher-than-tolerable numbers of complaints.

If they pay attention, organizations *can* determine during the hiring process whether a physician has the capacity to achieve high levels of patient satisfaction (Snyder 2016). Leaders often report that they saw signs of a physician's lack of ability in this area, only to hire him anyway because "we were desperate to hire; we'd been searching for so long that we lowered our standards."

If you're one of the physicians who has to work with the doctor who is unable to offer patients a satisfying encounter, you see the unfairness in this decision.

15. *Good team members are retained by "re-recruiting."* Leading organizations often have a formal process by which they reach out to high performers to let them know how much their efforts are appreciated. Their administrators also probe for issues that can be addressed to create a better work environment for doctors or help them become even more engaged. And they follow up on any issues the doctors raised the last time they met.

16. *Low performers are dealt with.* A group can raise its collective satisfaction scores if everyone improves *or* if low-scoring providers are replaced by higher-scoring ones. Unfortunately, many of the lowest performers don't improve on their own initiative. The best organizations don't ignore the problem; they wade in and deal with it.

Embedding patient engagement into physicians' performance expectations drives accountability, prevents unpleasant surprises, and makes the review process logical and objective. Most organizations have a formal performance review process; it's the improvement component that is too often left to chance.

High-performing organizations follow a consistent approach to dealing with low-scoring physicians, starting with informal and then more-formal conversations, moving to support and resources, and then invoking a progressive disciplinary process. Finally, having applied this system fairly, these organizations will be fully equipped to say to the physician, "It just isn't a good fit. We need to part ways."

Organizations that support doctors' efforts to improve their interactions with patients need not do all 16 things in this chapter to make a big impact. They typically start small, choosing one or two approaches to implement and then, once confirming success, expand to broader efforts. Many take an individualized approach (especially if they have just a few doctors who are really struggling) and make a thoughtful effort to add supports that create the best chance of success for each doctor.

But even if your organization provides none of this help or support, you can undertake improvement on your own. Take heart in the fact that while most physicians practice in an environment where some organizational support for improving patient satisfaction is provided, more help is usually desired.

If you have to take efforts mostly into your own hands, Chapter 7 tells you how to do it.

REFERENCES

Barnas, K. 2011. "ThedaCare's Business Performance System: Sustaining Continuous Daily Improvement Through Hospital Management in a Lean Environment." *Joint Commission Journal on Quality and Patient Safety* 37 (9): 387–99, AP1–AP8.

Snyder, B. 2016. *The Best Patient Experience: Helping Physicians Improve Care, Satisfaction, and Scores.* Chicago: Health Administration Press.

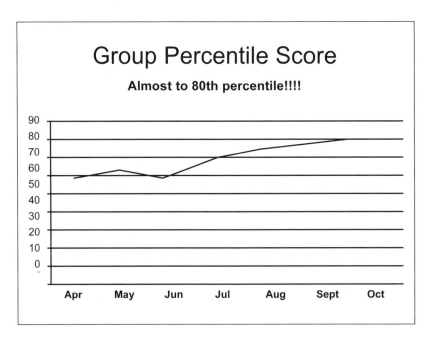

XYZ Physician Group
Patient Satisfaction Review
3rd Quarter

Group Percentile Score
Almost to 80th percentile!!!!

(continued)

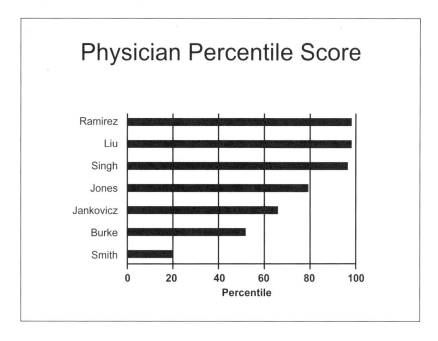

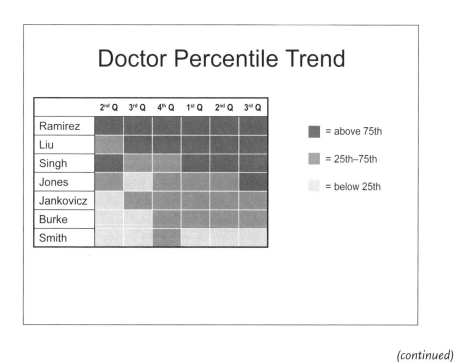

(continued)

(continued from previous page)

3rd Quarter Formal Complaints

- Rude/argumentative (3)

- Doctor was checking his cell phone (1)

- Wouldn't give me the medication I wanted (1)

3rd Quarter Feedback from Surveys
Representative Examples—Criticisms

- ". . . doctor seemed rushed . . ."

- "He took a call during our visit."

- "He left before I could ask my question. It's not that I'm slow, but I had to formulate my question. He blew out of the room before I could get my thoughts together. I was embarrassed to ask him to wait."

- "I never felt like I got a good explanation of what was causing my pain."

- "She wasn't too interested in what I had to say. I felt like she jumped to conclusions. They didn't all make sense based on what I had been experiencing. I might want to try a different doctor next time."

(continued)

(continued from previous page)

3rd Quarter Feedback from Surveys

Representative Examples—Kudos!

- "Dr. Singh is so nice. I just love him."

- "I know I'm a rambler. But Dr. Liu is so diplomatic when I get off track."

- "Dr. Ramirez knows I don't like to take medications if I can avoid them. He did a nice job explaining options and why going on the medication was a very good idea."

- "The doctor did a nice job explaining everything. He really listened to everything I told him and took it all into account."

- "Dr. Jankovicz is really a kind person. She always asks me about my grandkids."

Lightning Roundtable

In 30 seconds or less, share with the group the behavior you're currently working on to improve:

(continued)

(continued from previous page)

Deep Dive: Five Minutes

Today's deep dive is sharing strategies to redirect patients who want to share their life story when you've got a very busy schedule in front of you.

• Offer something that has worked for you
• Decide on next quarter's deep dive topic

Source: Snyder (2016).

CHAPTER 7

If You Have to Go It Alone

A FEW DOCTORS find themselves in a position of having to improve their interactions with patients *completely* on their own. And many more are caught in one of these scenarios:

- You're a doctor in an organization whose leaders understand that there's a problem (generally low patient satisfaction survey scores), so those leaders go around waving survey results and pointing fingers. They do not offer to be part of the solution, nor do they recognize that blaming others almost never fixes the problem—it usually just irritates folks and creates another problem.

- You're at a critical crossroads where your leader says, "You've got to do better or we'll need to part ways. If you'd like to stay, you've got to figure it out." The organization has not offered support to help you "figure it out."

- Your organization is getting better at offering support, but you're looking to advance your improvement farther and faster. You're impatient (good for you!). By experimenting with new concepts that could eventually be adopted by your organization, you could be a leader in this area—a catalyst for change that accelerates improvement.

The tools and insights in this chapter can help. Here, we take a look at the biggest obstacles for those who are going it alone (or mostly alone) and provide tips to address those challenges.

MAINTAINING MOTIVATION AND FOCUS

This is, by far, the most challenging issue for doctors who don't have the supporting organizational structure—such as regular meetings or scheduled reminder e-mails—to keep the issue front and center. Without that structure, your best intentions can easily get swept away by the whirlwind that takes over every minute of your day. You won't consciously decide to stop focusing on improving your interactions with patients, but it'll happen.

Instead, build your own structure with these straightforward tips for maintaining focus on both a daily or weekly basis and a monthly or quarterly basis.

Daily/Weekly Focus

Keeping the importance of positive patient interactions at the top of your mind is a great way to improve their overall quality. Several doctors I know have the discipline to pause for a micro-second before entering the patient's room and remind themselves of the importance of the interaction they're about to have. Give that a try, especially when you are tired or are getting ready to see a patient you know will be challenging.

Enlist support from others to help keep you focused on improving. Have colleagues and other members of the care team ask you in the hallway or break room, "Hey, what are you working on today?" When you reply, "Working on repeating key points the patient has told me" (for example), you've had a conversation that can reinforce spectacular results over time:

- It reminds you of the *one thing* you're working on and forces it back to top of mind.

- It forces you to give "public testimony" to your colleagues; if you don't follow through with what you're working on, you'll look undisciplined and risk minor embarrassment.

- It gets others involved. If someone hasn't asked you in a while, you can remind her with some good-natured ribbing. More so, it provides people you like and trust an opportunity to help you, and they'll like that.

- Importantly, it's an ultra-visible demonstration of your leadership in this area. Your effort may become contagious.

Put a five-minute appointment on your weekly calendar to reflect on the importance of having good interactions with patients and what skill or behavior you're currently working on. Or send a brief, weekly e-mail to a short list of people telling them what you're resolving to do better. This list can include colleagues, members of the team, your leader, your spouse, your kids, and so on. Or if you're really into brevity, tweet it! The exercise should take no longer than five minutes.

The point is to establish a routine so that you don't lose your focus and commitment. But it's also another way to establish yourself within your group as a leader on the subject.

Monthly/Quarterly Focus

To take stock of your efforts every month or quarter, keep a notebook or a folder on your tablet and write down what you've been working on, what your successes and challenges have been, and what you'll be working on next. If you have any data to show the results of your efforts, write those down, too.

Then complete or update your patient satisfaction scorecard and action plan (see Appendix 5.4). Don't have the survey data to fill in the first section? Simply move on to complete the strengths, opportunities for improvement, and monthly journal sections. I've also seen doctors do their journaling on a sheet of paper, note card, or sticky note. Be sure to post it in an eye-catching spot near your desk.

You can e-mail this monthly or quarterly journaling to your colleagues or support team. (Feel free to include me, at Bo@BoSnyderConsulting.com, with a quick report! A number of nonclients do this, and I enjoy hearing from them.)

Finally, if you adopt the "instant input" patient cards described in the next section, summarize what you've learned this month or quarter through this method of input as well.

KNOWING HOW WELL YOU'RE DOING

The second major challenge you'll have if you're going it alone is being able to occasionally take stock of how well your work is paying off. The best way to overcome this challenge is to

know your patient satisfaction survey data.

If you don't have access to those data, obtain your own.

Although all large healthcare organizations (and all hospitals, regardless of size) survey patients, some smaller organizations do not. And even if your organization does conduct a survey, there is no guarantee you'll be given the opportunity to see the responses about you specifically. Following are some guidelines for obtaining data on your own:

- *If your organization has patient satisfaction survey data, see it as your job to find them.* Work through your medical director to find out who "owns" the data. Become best friends with someone in that department. Ask for her help in accessing the data and explaining them to you. In fact, ask to see the actual survey; you want to be aware of what questions your patients are being asked. With her guidance, you can become an expert in how survey data should—and should not—be interpreted and used. If she can't answer your questions, ask that a call be scheduled for you to talk directly with a representative from the survey vendor.

- *Find out how to gain access to the verbatim patient comments about you from the patient satisfaction surveys.* This is where the patient gets to offer any feedback he chooses in free form. Sometimes this feedback is pure gold.

   Along this vein, also become friends with the people in the patient relations department who handle patient complaints. Let them know you'd like to see any comments related to you, and you'd like to see them as soon as possible after they are received. One hopes these folks would contact you anyway, but it's good to build a relationship with them and establish yourself as someone who takes feedback seriously.

- *Hand out "instant input" patient cards, such as the one shown in the box on the opposite page.* Make sure you have a clear understanding with staff about how the returned cards should be handled and how results should be compiled and reported to you. You may find that you'll have to do this on your own. If so, it will be worth the effort.

- *Check out public sources of feedback about yourself on websites such as Healthgrades.com and RateMD.com.* While these sites may have somewhat limited patient-comment content now, I expect them to become more used in the not-too-distant future. And more websites like them will spring up.

GUIDANCE ON WHERE TO FOCUS YOUR EFFORTS

My advice on what to do if you're going it alone is similar to what you'd do if you had organizational support: Identify a very short list of behavior changes that will have the biggest impact on the quality of your interactions with patients.

Instant Input Patient Cards

If your practice does not collect doctor-specific data on its patient satisfaction survey (or does not survey patients at all), here's a fast, inexpensive, and easy way to get input from *your* patients.

At the end of the visit, hand your patient a printed card (such as the one shown below), a pen, and an envelope labeled with only your name. As you present the card, you might say,

> I'd like to ask you to do me a favor. I am trying to improve how I interact with my patients. If you could just take 30 seconds to jot down the **one** *most important thing* you think I could do better, I would really appreciate it.

> Be really honest. You don't have to sign it! I won't know who it's from; I have a lot of patients today. You can just seal it in the envelope and leave it in the box at the front desk when you leave. Thanks! I really appreciate it.

Whether you review the cards yourself or have a staff member compile the responses for you, it will be worth the effort. What valuable input! And even if a patient chooses to not complete the card, what a great impression you've made: *"Wow, my doctor really cares what I think!"*

To improve how you interact with me—your patient—the ONE most important thing you could do differently is:

_____

_____

_____

As described in Chapter 5, to make that list, take a few minutes to complete a *self-assessment* (see Appendix 5.1). Take your time on this, be honest with yourself, and see it as an investment in your professional development. Also as part of this exercise, complete the *"where to start" worksheet* (Appendix 5.2). It allows you to rank the patient-interaction components that match up to the framework for engaging patients provided in Exhibit 1.1.

The self-assessment is most helpful if you review it in tandem with others' assessments of you. See the sample *staff and peer questionnaires* in Appendix 5.3. Asking your support staff or partners to give you their impressions of your strengths and weaknesses with patients can be eye-opening, humbling, uplifting—and surprising! Bite the bullet and find out what they think. Opening yourself to their input demonstrates your leadership, confidence, and maturity. Asking for their feedback may prompt others to examine their own patient interactions.

Another source of guidance is feedback from a *coach*, as discussed in Chapter 5. Often, doctors are willing to pay for a day of shadowing and coaching out of their own pocket. If this option isn't feasible for you, consider lobbying your employer to pay the fee in exchange for your commitment to improve. Another avenue is to solicit someone in your organization who has some coaching experience.

If you are reading this book, you are already motivated enough to move forward, even without support from your organization. And because motivation is key, you have every chance of being successful!

CHAPTER 8

Journeying to 99th Percentile Patient Satisfaction—One Group's Story

PATIENT SATISFACTION SCORES can improve rapidly—not just for individual doctors but for whole groups of doctors as well. Take the experience of an emergency medicine group that made incredible progress in just one year—and has sustained it since.

Imagine yourself as a member of this group. Would these experiences have helped you? What can you draw from this case study that you can apply to your situation regardless of what your group is doing—or not doing? Key insights are highlighted at the end of the chapter.

THE PRACTICE

First Physician Corporation (FPC) is a privately owned physician group. It employs 11 emergency medicine physicians and 15 mid-level providers who see patients exclusively at Charlton Memorial Hospital in Fall River, Massachusetts.

Fall River is a coastal community located near the Rhode Island state line. It is predominately blue collar with a large Portuguese-speaking population. The community is served by one other hospital.

More than 70,000 patient visits occur each year in the Charlton emergency department (ED), with about 40 percent of those served through a fast-track urgent care model staffed by the mid-level providers—physician assistants and nurse practitioners.

FPC has always been proud of its stability and the quality of its providers. Many have been with the group for a decade or more.

FPC'S PAST PATIENT SATISFACTION RESULTS

For years, the group focused on providing good care, efficiently delivered. It tracked the performance indicators common for emergency medicine providers: patients seen per hour, patients returning to the ED within 72 hours, admission rates, rates of mortality or transfer to the intensive care unit within 24 hours, and adherence to Centers for Medicare & Medicaid Services quality measures.

The group didn't pay much attention to patient satisfaction scores, which weren't great. FPC's level of awareness changed in 2010 when Charlton's competitor was acquired by a private equity firm. The new owner soon announced a capital infusion that would result in significant facility upgrades in the competitor's ED and a strategic focus on increasing ED market share.

In no position to match those facility upgrades, the leaders at Charlton quickly zeroed in on the poor patient satisfaction scores in the ED. What had been a non-issue suddenly came into sharp focus as both a problem and an opportunity.

Charlton's senior leadership asked FPC to improve its patient satisfaction scores as a part of the broader effort to improve the scores for the ED as a whole. Much discussion ensued, both between the group and hospital and among FPC doctors. The doctors knew they had to embrace the hospital's challenge; because the group gets paid for each patient it treats, the providers' livelihood was at stake.

"My personal patient satisfaction scores were among the lowest in the group," says Brian Tsang, MD, FPC president (personal communication, November 5, 2014). "And that helped me convince the group to accept this shift in priorities, because anything I asked them to do, I was going to have to do, too."

On this and other efforts, Tsang works in partnership with Lissa B. Singer, NP, CPC-I, the group's chief quality officer. She notes (personal communication, November 13, 2014), "It was important for us to show the hospital that we were in the game, committed, and serious about improvement. Patient satisfaction is just one of our improvement initiatives, but once things started moving in a positive direction, it became really hard to *not* want that continued success."

Tsang made one key request of Charlton's leaders: The hospital must invest in obtaining a larger sampling of ED patients for its patient satisfaction survey. With a larger sampling, each provider could get a more convincing, and more statistically reliable, number of patient survey responses each quarter. This critical mass added to the credibility of individual scores.

MAKING DECISIONS AND GAINING MOMENTUM

Through the spring and summer of 2012, FPC decided how to proceed. It took a while, and that was good.

"We're very democratic," Tsang says. "That means things take a little more time, but the final decisions have more buy-in. And I know that the best ideas don't come from me. The group will eventually make a good decision if you let people participate and give it some time."

Interestingly, before its first ideas were implemented, the group's patient satisfaction scores already began to climb. Simply raising awareness of the issue prompted the doctors to make subtle changes in the ways they engaged with patients.

FPC started its improvement journey by providing the following educational materials to each member:

- Slides from an emergency medicine conference presentation on improving patient satisfaction
- Improvement tips from the group's patient satisfaction survey vendor
- A recent article on patient satisfaction from *Consumer Reports* that included scores from Massachusetts doctors

And the group made several key decisions:

- Each provider would receive his or her individual patient satisfaction scores by e-mail along with the scores of every other provider in the group. When this process began, the peer data were blinded. In other words, each provider knew his or her scores and the scores of everyone else in the group, but not to whom each of those other scores belonged.
- Six months later, the group decided to unblind individual provider names when these results were reported. Everyone would know exactly how they stacked up against everyone else.

  Scary, right? No! The providers saw this as a natural evolution. In fact, it caused a great deal of discussion among providers about the results and how some in the group were able to achieve higher scores. Tsang emphasizes that the scores weren't seen as measures of the providers' value as human beings but merely as another important measure of performance.
- The doctors came to realize that the initial educational materials they received, while helpful, didn't go far enough. So they interviewed outside coaches who could provide one-on-one shadow coaching and facilitate group conversations about especially challenging issues.

Importantly, the group never lost sight of the big picture. The cross-town competitor was threatening the entire Charlton ED, and the FPC doctors understood their role in helping the ED improve the patient experience. Tsang notes:

We had to take ownership of what we could do to address the problem. Our ED was facing a new competitive threat. And if we didn't respond, our livelihood could be threatened.

It was tempting to play the role of the victim and blame the hospital and its ED staff who had at least as much room for improvement as our group did. We decided we had to fix our own house first. We knew that the reason patients come to the ED is to see the doctor. If we could improve that part of the experience, overall scores for the total experience might rise, and we would have caused that to happen through our efforts.

The other benefit of making headway on our own performance is that we could show the rest of the ED team that it could be done. We could be the role model. They couldn't credibly make excuses once we had proven it could be done.

We worked with the hospital ED staff to support them and reinforce positive behaviors, but the most important thing we did was to get our own house in order.

FPC doctors began to work with ED staff on basic scripting and raising awareness. Two early examples were making sure that staff never left patients without inquiring about their comfort and always greeting patients upon arrival with, "Welcome to Charlton. How can I help you?"

COACHING INTERVENTION

In September 2012, the group brought me in as a coach to spend a week with them, mostly one-on-one with individual providers. The group's "naturals"—those who were born patient interaction superstars—received little coaching time, perhaps one or two hours each. Most "typical" providers received two to four hours of shadowing and coaching, depending on their past patient satisfaction scores.

I gave each provider immediate, individual feedback on his or her strengths and opportunities for improvement. In collaboration with me, each provider identified a short list of key changes he or she could make to improve interactions with patients.

Some immediately began practicing their "single most important change" while I watched and provided support. All received a written report summarizing key strengths, a prioritized list of change opportunities, and goals. Appendix 8.1, at the end of this chapter, provides examples of my comments regarding strengths and weaknesses.

As part of the coaching process, I also facilitated small discussion groups—structured but informal gatherings that gave the providers a chance to review the data, ask questions, brainstorm solutions to common problems, and learn from each other. These conversations deepened the doctors' understanding of the issues and strengthened their commitment to taking the next steps on their personal improvement journeys.

POST-COACHING ACCELERATION

To maximize and leverage the impact of their investment in shadow coaching, the doctors looked for opportunities to hardwire what they'd learned. One especially effective practice was a quarterly "confessional."

This process, carried out via e-mail with lots of back-and-forth among the providers, asked people to articulate their key opportunities for improvement, what they were doing to improve, and what their successes had been. The expectation was that everyone, even those best at interacting with patients, would identify a personal challenge and work on it.

Tsang says, "We wanted to normalize the topic of patient satisfaction by sharing 'tricks of the trade'—just like we do for technical stuff like pediatric sedation or shoulder dislocations. And we wanted to create a sense that we were all here to help each other improve."

The process also instilled some subtle, helpful peer pressure. It reminded each provider about the one or two very important things he or she should be working on and encouraged follow-through and accountability to improve. Furthermore, it kept everyone's awareness level high.

Soon, individuals' competitiveness and humor began to emerge, with providers playfully teasing and encouraging one another.

"We were careful to keep it constructive, but there was always some trash-talking and strutting when the scores came out. After all, we have been getting test scores for our whole lives," Tsang says. "We had a good time with it. And it helped us to always be thinking about our interactions with patients." Examples of providers' confessional comments are provided in Appendix 8.2.

The confessionals process was repeated quarterly. Providers reported on progress and moved on to other challenges once initial gains had been made.

Soon, FPC providers emerged as credible leaders on patient satisfaction improvement, and they leveraged this credibility by engaging the ED nursing staff to support them in their efforts. For example, they began giving kudos to nurses who went above and beyond the call of duty with patients. And staff members who provided great service were entered into a drawing for an iPad several times each year, courtesy of the group.

99TH PERCENTILE—AND SUSTAINING IT!

At the close of the fourth quarter of 2012, FPC had collected enough patient surveys to reveal an accurate picture of improvement. When the doctors saw that their scores had reached the 99th percentile, their pride was palpable, and their credibility within Charlton Hospital and with the other members of the ED staff was sky high. Exhibit 8.1 shows the improvement trends for the group. Exhibits 8.2 and 8.3 show how individual physician scores improved.

   To its credit, the group immediately recognized the importance of sustaining this remarkable achievement. Today, three key approaches help the FPC physicians to do just that:

1. *The group monitors and reports overall patient satisfaction scores quarterly.* Any significant or sustained decrease serves as a warning to consider reinstating other approaches, such as the confessionals, which have been replaced by a mentoring program that pairs underperforming physicians with a high-performing peer for four hours of shadowing.

Exhibit 8.1: First Physician Corporation Patient Satisfaction Percentile Score, Group Composite

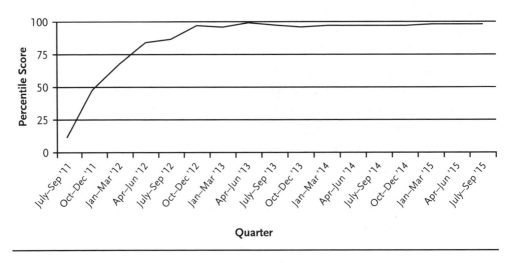

Source: First Physician Corporation and Southcoast Hospitals Group.

Exhibit 8.2: 2011 First Physician Corporation Patient Satisfaction Percentile Score, by Provider

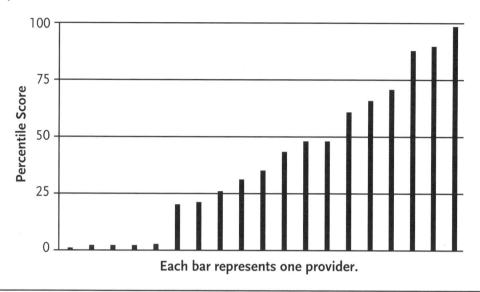

Each bar represents one provider.

Source: First Physician Corporation and Southcoast Hospitals Group.

Exhibit 8.3: 2015 First Physician Corporation Patient Satisfaction Percentile Score, by Provider

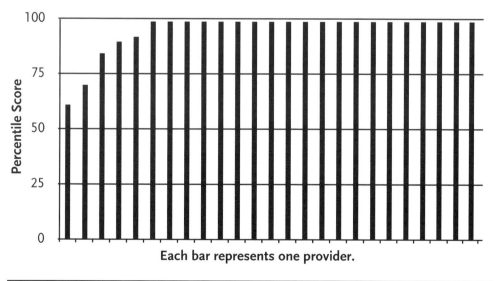

Each bar represents one provider.

Source: First Physician Corporation and Southcoast Hospitals Group.

2. *Unblinded, provider-specific scores are published quarterly.* Each provider is never more than three months away from having his or her performance revealed to peers. This makes it impossible to hide or free-ride on the efforts of colleagues.

3. *Any provider whose scores fall below the 75th percentile in a quarter must undergo mentoring through the peer-mentorship program.* Those with scores above the 90th percentile are asked to become mentors. Underperforming mentees do not get paid for their time in this session, while mentors are paid a bonus for their assistance. Typically, just a handful of providers are mentored each quarter, as you can see in Exhibit 8.3.

"OWNERSHIP" FOR EMPLOYED PHYSICIANS

"How do we get our doctors to behave like yours do?"

This is the question Tsang gets when he speaks at conferences. FPC physicians did have one significant advantage on their journey: Because they are part of a private group, they *own themselves.* "Owning"—whether in the literal sense (as with a private group) or in a figurative sense (as in taking ownership)—is often the difference between placing at the 30th percentile and the 97th.

But even if you are an employee, you are still president, CEO, and chairman of the board of Dr. You, Inc. By owning your improvement, you enhance your brand, your potential success in the employment market, and—importantly—your job satisfaction.

SUMMARY OF KEY POINTS AND INSIGHTS

If you have taken ownership and recognize a need to improve, you can take advantage of these insights from FPC's experience:

- It is easier to improve if you do it with others. Take advantage of group opportunities if they are available. If they are not, advocate for them or find one or two motivated colleagues to join you.

- Improvement can happen in a short amount of time after years of lagging scores.

- Merely raising awareness of the issue can prompt you to make subtle changes that improve patient satisfaction scores.

- Be thoughtful about how to proceed, and you'll avoid hasty decisions and false starts.
- Getting individual, statistically reliable satisfaction survey data for *each doctor's* patients is crucial.
- Your progress will be more rapid if your patient satisfaction data are shown to your colleagues, and vice versa. Subtle peer pressure works.
- An outside coach can be helpful, especially if you then make the most of the information received in the shadow-coaching experience.
- You can make this fun! FPC capitalized on the esprit de corps and playfulness among its members as they supported each other on their improvement journeys.

Appendix 8.1 Examples of My Comments to FPC Physicians Following Shadow Coaching

Examples of Strength Comments

"Very nice job of putting the chest pain patient at ease. He was very anxious, and you made his anxiety go away just by explaining how you were going to run some tests to rule out the potentially serious causes."

"You connected with all your patients almost immediately. You greeted them all by name."

"You always paused before leaving the exam bay and asked if they had any questions or if anything was unclear. Very nice job."

"You always took a few extra seconds to share your clinical thinking with each patient. They understood the 'why' behind everything you did. They appreciated that, and as a result they had very few questions for you."

"You made a point to say goodbye to that lady as they were transporting her upstairs. She was so pleased to hear that. And she sincerely thanked you for your help."

Examples of Opportunity Comments

"When you have to leave the room for just a minute to get supplies, remember to tell the patient why you're leaving and that you'll be right back. Don't make them guess why you're leaving or how long you'll be gone."

(continued)

(continued from previous page)

"Always say goodbye, wish them well, and shake their hand."

"You left the room several times without asking for questions. One time the patient's family member shouted a question at you as you were leaving. Remember to pause and ask for questions before you leave."

"Slow down—especially when you first meet a patient. Take a moment to build a rapport before beginning to rattle off your questions."

"Nice job with that elderly patient with many medical problems. The only suggestion I have is to pause toward the end of your interaction and summarize your main points and what's going to happen next. There were a lot of things going on with her, and I'm not sure she totally understood everything that was happening."

Appendix 8.2 Confessionals Allowed Feedback and Support

Providers at First Physician Corporation used group e-mail to share progress reports about the behavior changes each was working on. Their comments* were insightful, funny, and sometimes both. Many reflect the providers being critical of themselves and their low scores. (These confessionals were generated by the group before its scores had seen much improvement.)

Would you be comfortable sharing thoughts like these with your colleagues?

> *"OK, my numbers are terrible. I am not sure what happened. Most likely I reverted to my quickness, less time in room. One comment was 'minimized what happened.' So going forward I will TOTALLY empathize with the 1/4 inch cut, bump on shin, and cold × 2 days!"*

> *"I do find that explaining all the work that goes into telling a patient that it's safe to go home is typically better received than, 'Well, everything looks great!' That reassurance typically falls flat no matter how true it may be. Going through the battery of tests performed validates the wait and the copay. Takes some time but I think it's well worth it."*

*Some identifying details have been omitted.   *(continued)*

(continued from previous page)

"My scores suck this time around, but I don't think they are accurate! Anyhoo, I agree that people enjoy a jovial attitude at times. Also I think that buttering up the family helps the survey scores because they probably help the patient fill the survey out eventually."

"My thing has been to validate the patients coming in for evaluation into the ED. I tell them that everything we have done as a cursory check in the ER was normal, but I let them know that I truly believe they are having pain or are sick and that their search for a reason shouldn't end in the ER. Our job is to rule out an emergency condition that requires immediate intervention. I stress the need for them to follow up with their PCP to continue to search for an answer. Patients seem to be ok with a lack of a definitive diagnosis once I have explained our role."

"I get the patient's name before I go in, so I can address them by name from the start. I like going in without a chart in hand, but then I don't have the name unless I make a point of getting it. I already introduce myself to all family members, but I am going to start to ask them for their names too. I have done this a few times, and I forget their names almost immediately, but they seem to appreciate it. And it helps slow me down."

"I ask if there are any questions prior to leaving the room. Sometimes I forget but go back into the room as soon as I realize this and say 'I'm sorry but I neglected to ask if you have any questions at this time.'"

"What is working for me: letting the patient finish talking completely. Even count to five to make sure they are finished before I start asking questions. Getting water, lots of water, and box lunches. Having more fun with patients, even if they don't seem in the mood to laugh—they usually do. What I am going to try to do: try again to sit down. Drag a stool in or a trash can if necessary. Bring water for family members. Go over discharge instructions before the nurse gives them. I was good at first about thanking them for choosing us—I need to start that again. I have been printing out x-rays for fractures—that works so well that I think I will try printing even normal ones."

"It's hard to tell you everything I do because honestly, I change my tactic based on the patient. I try to read my audience. Some people want humor.

(continued)

(continued from previous page)

Some people want empathy. Some people want me to agree that the world really is out to get them and everything bad ever only happens to them. My only tactics that are consistent are: (1) Smiling. I realize that I am a smiler by nature and that others might find this difficult but I think it helps my scores. People frequently comment on how 'nice' or 'friendly' I am. . . And I believe it's because I smile a lot. It's just a perception. (2) Giving the patient a plan. With every patient, after I get my hx and perform my PE, I tell them the plan."

"The biggest thing I try and do for every patient, especially the ones being discharged, is go back into the room and 'wrap it up,' answer any last minute questions. Even people without a diagnosis appreciate this, at least I tried to find out what was causing the 5 years of pelvic pain."

"I do realize that I speak quickly and have incorporated a few things that have FORCED me to slow down when I speak. I have paused in the middle and at the end, and admitted to them that I speak quickly and asked at least 2 times if I can clarify anything better. Since they often remember only some of what we say, this gives them a minute to digest things in smaller pieces."

"I have noticed the patient and family members in the room are shocked when you thank them for coming in. Or if I say, 'Please don't hesitate to return with any worsening symptoms or any new problems.' They appreciate that."

"I am now working on the discharge portion of the encounter as I realized 2 or 3 times last week I discharged patients and got caught up in something and they were gone before I got back in. When appropriate (and I know already they will be going home), I will stop in as tests are coming back and say something like: 'I may not see you again before you are discharged so I'll say goodbye now. It was a pleasure meeting you. Hope you feel better soon.'"

"I have forgotten to greet the patients with their name when it is very busy, so I must get back to that. Maybe that's why my doctor courtesy score dropped. I am going to try and thank the pt. for coming to see us at the end of the visit. Maybe last impressions will revive my scores!!"

(continued)

(continued from previous page)

"I can honestly report to the group that I pause before starting my physical exam (and actually request permission to do so) over 90% of the time. People seem to respond well to this. It does slow me down somewhat, as I used to start examining people while I was still asking them questions."

"One thing I think is helping me is that I am less afraid to make people laugh. Even if they are really sick, it is not that hard; they are an easy audience, and laugh at pretty lame jokes. They also don't seem to be offended."

"I have taken some of your suggestions and begun addressing everybody in the room. Patients and their families seem to respond very well to this."

"I am trying to make sure I do the 'middle' visit, to give a progress report. I try to do this right after I see an x-ray or CT—then say we are just waiting for labs. I never liked going in until I was sure their symptoms had been treated (nausea, pain, etc.) but too often I would forget. If I do forget, and realize everything is back but I haven't gone in yet, I will even cheat! Meaning I will go in, ask how they are, say we are still waiting for one result, then go back in 5 minutes later after I've finished the discharge paperwork to tell them the final results."

"When the ER is busy, and we are way behind, I am trying to pop in a room right next to the one I just saw to say 'still waiting on results.' The month of October, I threw it on very thick to the patients. I will be interested to see my new survey results to see if I need to completely change again or reach out for more help."

"I make a tactile gesture prior to breaking ties for this round with either a hand on the shoulder, handshake, caress of the cheek, sometimes a peck for the elderly ladies; and, of course I thank them. . . Yeah, and what if this whole time my gentle caress of the elderly woman's face was construed as cheap flirtation by her spouse!" [Author's note: Just to be clear, this provider was having fun with his colleagues.]

"My recent scores must be wrong, I thought I was perfect? It must be a character flaw of this community." [Author: More fun.]

"I agree there are time limits to my smiling. It's 2:15 a.m. and it's my third back pain. The patient has had the chronic pain for months but decided

(continued)

(continued from previous page)

to come in at this hour for repair. I used to get upset and shake my head, but I seem to be trending towards pulling up a chair, laughing inside, and smiling."

"Although my recent survey score is less than admirable this time around, I have tried implementing a time estimate of testing. I thought this was a good idea because it gives patients and their family a rough idea of how long they'll be in the ER. It may backfire if it takes way longer than expected, but in general, I get the sense that patients and family appreciate the time estimates. I may need to resort to carrying warm blankets if the scores don't go up next time!"

"This has made a difference with my personal job satisfaction, I find my day dominated with positive interactions and not 'me against them' type of interactions. I'm looking forward to my next round of scores. I don't know what I'll do if my scores are lower, but I'm sure one of you can prescribe me something to at least make me feel good!"

Part IV

FOR SKEPTICS

CHAPTER 9

A Dozen Reasons You Should Care About Patient Satisfaction

IF YOU'RE READING this book of your own accord, you probably think being appreciated by your patients is a good thing. But have you thought about all the reasons it's important?

If you're like me, your top-of-mind reason that doctors should provide a great patient experience is that it's the right thing to do. You have uniquely intimate relationships with human beings who are sick, scared, and vulnerable. Being respectful to them should be a no-brainer.

But for some doctors, it's not. I've heard plenty who have low scores make statements such as, "I just don't think satisfaction is that important."

Certainly, how satisfied or engaged a patient is with her experience is determined by a complex set of factors, including processes and supporting structure in the healthcare setting. *But interaction with the provider is the key driver.* No surprise there: You are in the driver's seat.

Author Stephen Beeson, MD, in his book *Practicing Excellence,* makes excellent arguments in favor of the notion that physicians should care deeply about the patient experience (Beeson 2006). His rationale for "the case for service" got me thinking about even more reasons—12 in all—why doctors should embrace the importance of patient satisfaction.

CLASSIC REASONS

These reasons for caring about patient satisfaction have been around forever, or at least since medicine entered the modern era 100 years ago.

Reflection: How Important Is Patient Satisfaction to You?

Consider each of the indicators of success below and ask yourself,

"How important is this to me?"

"What am I doing to manage this area?"

"How well am I doing in this area?"

"How do I know?"

Being a good clinician	Being financially successful
Being safe from litigation	Being appreciated by my patients
Having collegiality with my partners	Making good use of my time
Growing my practice	Staying current and innovating

There is no optimal way to rank these indicators. Every physician is different—as is every practice. And certainly each component is integral to success.

But you'll find it valuable to spend a few minutes reflecting on where patient satisfaction fits among your other priorities. The fact that it should *be* a priority is a given.

Reason 1. Bottom Line, Healthcare Really Is About Caring

This is my best response to a doctor who says, "We have more important things to worry about." Wrong! Stellar clinical skills won't be appreciated if the patient feels you've asked questions brusquely or rushed his exam. His most basic expectation—that his doctor would care about him—was not met.

Let me be direct: If a doctor isn't appreciated by the vast majority of his patients, he is not a good doctor.

After all, "caring" is what our industry exists to do. Most physicians understand this, and many embrace it—they became doctors precisely because they care about others.

On the other hand, the reason you became a doctor really doesn't matter. It may be significant to *you*, but not necessarily to your patients nor to their families. Their universal *expectation* is that you chose to practice medicine because you care.

Reason 2. Be Nice or You'll Lose Them

How you interact with a patient now determines whether you'll have a chance to interact with that patient—or with her neighbors, coworkers, or Facebook friends—in the future. You must treat patents well or they won't come back, and they certainly won't recommend you to others.

To this point, Beeson (2006) cites a telling Harris poll published in *The Wall Street Journal* in 2004: People place more importance on doctors' interpersonal skills than on their medical judgment or experience, and doctors' failings in these areas are the overwhelming factor that drives patients to switch doctors.

More than a decade later, it's truer than ever. Take the experience of one of my client groups. Wanting to grow, its leaders tried outreach, advertising, joining new managed care networks—none of it made much of a difference. But when the group began to focus on delivering a great experience for its patients, it soon had a new problem: managing growth!

The group's volume swelled because far fewer patients left and more new patients showed up through word-of-mouth referrals, which are accelerated today—the age of social media. The foundation of patient loyalty is the relationship patients have with their doctor. Loyal patients don't say, "I'm going to see *the* doctor." They say, "I'm going to see *my* doctor."

Reason 3. Malpractice Risk Drops

Cited over and over again in the literature, the fact is, a doctor's relationship with her patients has a high correlation with whether they will sue her for malpractice.

Doctors who typically make an effort to partner with their patients, explain options and risks, communicate details, and make sure all questions are answered tend not to be sued. These doctors build credibility as skilled and caring people, and in general, patients are less likely to sue individuals they appreciate and respect.

NEWER REASONS

These reasons have emerged more recently and are in a state of flux. They relate mainly to ways publicly available patient satisfaction survey data are being used to compare healthcare providers.

Reason 4. Centers for Medicare & Medicaid Services Surveys Have Created More Transparency

In the past decade, the Hospital Consumer Assessment of Healthcare Providers and Systems (HCAHPS) and the more recently developed Clinician and Group Consumer Assessment of Healthcare Providers and Systems (CG-CAHPS) surveys have empowered comparison shoppers with new sources of information.

Until patient surveys became a part of the healthcare landscape a few decades ago, the patient experience was measured subjectively. And you didn't pay the price for patient dissatisfaction unless it caused significant and protracted word-of-mouth grousing.

No more. Hospital-specific patient satisfaction information is now available in all its objective glory for those who seek it. Beginning in 2008, hospitals are required to post patient satisfaction results on Hospital Compare's public website (www.hospitalcompare.hhs.gov) or face a financial penalty in Medicare reimbursement. By 2012, those patient satisfaction results were a part of the Centers for Medicare & Medicaid Services (CMS 2015) value-based purchasing formula to reward or penalize hospitals.

And office-specific data are on the way. Currently, CG-CAHPS is being piloted, just as HCAHPS was a decade ago. At the time of this writing, CMS has plans to begin pay-for-reporting schemes for certain large medical groups (AHRQ 2015). Expect that requirement to eventually extend to smaller physician group practices.

The private sector is following suit, with major insurers including patient satisfaction levels in their reimbursement formulas. Expect most payment systems to include patient satisfaction as a factor in physician reimbursement in coming years.

Reason 5. Everyone Likes Recognition and Awards—Both Winning Them and Telling Everyone

Patient satisfaction vendors are getting into the evaluation act by giving awards to the highest-scoring organizations. For example, National Research Corporation (NRC 2016) recognizes the nation's top hospitals with its Consumer Choice Awards each year. NRC fields a survey of more than 270,000 households to rate the hospitals in each market. The results are published, and the highest-ranking organizations in each community often promote themselves as award winners.

Imagine a future where the top medical groups (and individual doctors) in a community are recognized for their scores on private and government-sponsored satisfaction surveys. Imagine no more; that future is nearly here. CMS has begun to publish some physician-specific quality scores (Evans 2015). It's not a stretch to see the day when physician-specific patient satisfaction scores are published publicly. Those doctors who score well will absolutely use that information to promote themselves—not great news for everyone else.

Information companies such as Healthgrades.com and RateMDs.com don't give out awards, but an ever-increasing percentage of the public knows it can become better informed about healthcare services with a few mouse clicks. That's all it takes to see past patients' comments about specific doctors. If you're unfamiliar with those websites, log on to see what patients are saying about you.

Reason 6. Financial Risk and Reward: Value-Based Purchasing

Although we touched on this subject earlier in the chapter, the advent of value-based purchasing deserves its own place on this list.

So when exactly did hospital chief financial officers (CFOs) begin to care about patient satisfaction? When Medicare launched its Hospital Value-Based Purchasing program, a system of risk and reward in which a percentage of Medicare reimbursements to hospitals is put at risk based on performance on clinical quality and patient satisfaction. All of a sudden, CFOs started paying attention.

Some hospitals now receive more money than they otherwise would have. Some get less. In either case, they notice.

One benefit to the program is, no more guesswork! For the first time, at least to some degree, the financial impact of patient satisfaction performance can be objectively determined.

What does this mean for you? It means that your boss and your boss's boss want to know how you stack up on patient satisfaction. If you do an excellent job, you may be paid a retention bonus. If you drag scores down—or refuse to take the issue seriously, or fail to try to improve—you may be asked to seek employment elsewhere.

Reason 7. Social Media Are Here—and Growing

Never before have patients had the ability to share an unhappy experience at the doctor's office with hundreds of friends, neighbors, and coworkers at lightning speed—maybe while they're still in the exam room. A single disparaging tweet or Facebook post could be devastating to your practice. Patients see doctors when they're discouraged, angry, in pain, confused, and exhausted. Your behavior during their encounter can easily determine whether they leave the visit satisfied or bent on putting you out of business.

FIVE MORE REASONS YOU MAY NOT HAVE CONSIDERED

Reason 8. Higher Satisfaction Translates to Better Patient Compliance

The extent to which patients benefit from the course of treatment you've prescribed is directly related to how precisely they follow your advice. Whether it's taking their medications or rehabbing correctly after a total knee replacement, their choices post-visit or post-discharge affect the clinical outcomes for which you are responsible. This is not news to you, I'm sure.

Fortunately, you can influence how well your patients comply. It requires thoughtful communication, taking the time to explain your clinical thinking, and outlining what could happen if recommendations aren't followed.

Taking those steps will build a stronger relationship with your patients. They won't want to disappoint you—a caring person whom they trust and respect—by not following your instructions.

Reason 9. You Wield Power and Influence

As highly trained professionals in short supply, doctors carry enormous clout. But doctors who do their jobs in exceptional ways earn *the most* power and influence in their organizations, whether at large hospitals, group practices, or smaller physician offices. They lead by example. Their opinions are sought.

If you have great scores, staff will listen to you. You'll be known for being "great with patients." You will become an even more rarefied commodity than your peers.

Reason 10. You Experience More Pride in and Satisfaction with Your Job

This is a recurring theme among my clients. When they move the needle on their patient satisfaction scores, they're on top of the world. At work, they aren't merely applying their intellect or clinical skill set; they're making a significant impact on the lives of people who need help.

These physicians have the highest degree of satisfaction any professional could have. They respond to people in need and are worshipped by them. Be one of these lucky folks.

Reason 11. You Are Making Your Family Proud

That glow of pride and satisfaction radiates out to moms and uncles and other family members: *"My son is the best doctor in the world. He is smart as a whip. But he's also a great person whose patients rave about him. He really makes a difference."*

What a great reason to care about patient satisfaction, all on its own!

Reason 12. Better Relationships (and Reduced Turnover) Emerge Among Colleagues and Staff

Professionals who have great relationships with their customers create a positive workplace—an environment that attracts and keeps other energetic, like-minded people. An environment characterized by positive patient interactions cuts down on the cost and upheaval of staff and provider turnover. It also nurtures collaboration, which contributes to personal satisfaction. In other words, you'll stay happy and your coworkers will, too.

FOR THE UNCONVINCED

It won't surprise you that some doctors are unmoved by these arguments. Maybe you're one of them, or maybe you work with someone who is. I've heard enough objections to the need to focus on patient satisfaction to fill a book—or at least a chapter of a book. Many of them—and my responses—wound up in Chapter 10.

REFERENCES

Agency for Healthcare Research and Quality (AHRQ). 2015. "Clinician & Group." Accessed February 18, 2016. https://cahps.ahrq.gov/Surveys-Guidance/CG/index.html.

Beeson, S. C. 2006. "Individual Physician Coaching." Chap. 8 in *Practicing Excellence: A Physician's Manual to Exceptional Health Care*. Gulf Breeze, FL: Fire Starter Publishing.

Centers for Medicare & Medicaid Services (CMS). 2015. "Hospital Value-Based Purchasing." Updated October 30. www.cms.gov/Medicare/Quality-Initiatives-Patient-Assessment-Instruments/hospital-value-based-purchasing/index.html?redirect=/hospital-value-based-purchasing/.

Evans, M. 2015. "Providers Struggle on CMS Quality Measures." *Modern Healthcare*. Published December 12. www.modernhealthcare.com/article/20151212/MAGAZINE/312129964/providers-struggle-on-cms-quality-measures.

National Research Corporation (NRC). 2016. "Consumer Choice Awards." Accessed February 18. www.nationalresearch.com/about/consumer-choice-awards.

CHAPTER 10

Hard-to-Argue-With Responses to Common Objections

SOME DOCTORS REFLEXIVELY object when I suggest that they may be able to improve their interactions with patients. Self-assessment and behavior change are hard, especially if your typical day is spent on roller skates, tolerating frequent interruptions and making life-and-death decisions.

Perhaps you already understand the need to have good relationships with your patients and high patient satisfaction scores; it's only human to object every once in a while, even if only with the voice inside your head. Or maybe you're dealing with a colleague who's stuck. Here we discuss some common objections and helpful responses.

TYPICAL OBJECTIONS

I'm Already Doing Just Fine

Often this objection is unspoken, but it's there. And when I shadow physicians, I find that between one-third and one-half of them really *are* doing a good job interacting with their patients.

But others focus too much on "getting the job done," whether that's providing good clinical quality or seeing an enormous caseload. They often lack self-awareness and don't try to understand and meet the individual needs of each patient.

If you're one of these physicians, you must redefine "doing fine."

Ask yourself:

- Given that most patients won't tell you directly that they're dissatisfied, how do you know you're doing fine in their eyes?

- Do your patient satisfaction scores support your assessment? What about patient complaints?
- Do the nurses or your medical assistant ever compliment you on your bedside manner?
- Have you invited an impartial person to observe your interactions and offer an assessment and some feedback? Staff and colleagues know which doctors interact well with patients but may be uncomfortable giving negative feedback. So you need either performance data (survey results) or an assessment by an objective third party to determine whether you're really doing fine.

My Productivity Will Suffer

Physicians often assume that the magic answer to better patient engagement is to spend more time with each patient. And they don't know where they can find that time. To be fair, you often can't.

Consider this:

- Most groups have highly productive doctors who also have good patient satisfaction scores. They've figured out a way to make it work, and you can, too. Based on my experiences with many physician groups, Exhibit 10.1 demonstrates how productivity relates to patient satisfaction in a matrix format. When individual doctors are plotted in this way, there is always someone who scores highly on both.
- If improved productivity is your goal, you can achieve it without depriving patients of time with you. Talk to some of your more productive colleagues who also get high patient satisfaction scores. Time with their physician is what patients deserve.
- Doctors can no longer choose maximizing productivity *or* patient satisfaction. The new realities in healthcare require you to focus on productivity *and* patient satisfaction (and of course the technical aspects of quality care, too). Some of my clients have found that by trading just a *little bit* of productivity, they can improve their satisfaction scores significantly. Exhibit 10.2 shows this relationship in graph form.
- Patient satisfaction is one factor already affecting income—or it soon will be.
- Note that having higher-quality interactions with your patients won't necessarily require more time. A classic example is being aware of not allowing your patients to *perceive* that you're in a hurry.

Exhibit 10.1: Productivity–Patient Satisfaction Matrix

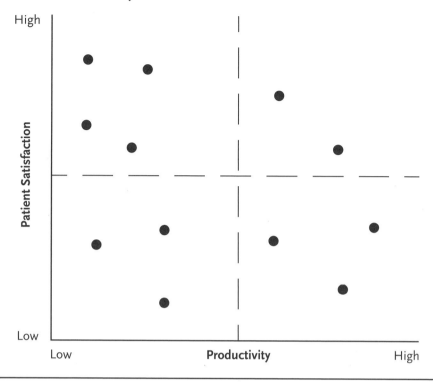

Note: Each dot represents a physician.

Exhibit 10.2: A Small Sacrifice in Productivity Results in a Large Gain in Patient Satisfaction

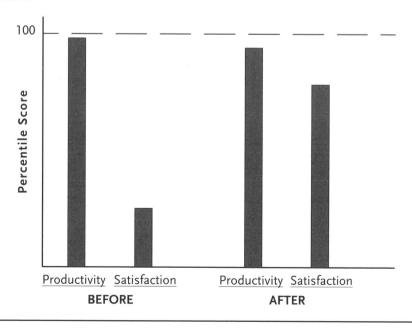

A Broad Response to a Physician Who Raises Every Objection

A blog post on KevinMD.com is from a disgruntled physician, lamenting hospitals' preoccupation with patient satisfaction scores (BirdStrike, MD 2013). As of this writing, the post was shared more than 16,000 times.

It essentially raises every objection covered in this chapter. In this sidebar, I share how I'd respond if I were the boss of a doctor who passionately raised the same complaint. I do this in case you are the doctor who wrote that blog post, or if you work with that doctor.

- I understand that the job of a physician is difficult and the field has changed a lot since you entered it. Venting is OK, even helpful, to cope with frustration. If you vent in your journal, that's fine. If you vent to me, that's fine, too. But please do not vent to your peers in our organization in an attempt to persuade them to your point of view.

- Scientists of behavior change management point out that some people have a hard time accepting change even after most people have accepted it and moved forward. This is normal. As long as you aren't contributing to negativity in the work environment, I won't hold your frustrations against you.

- Are you working on doing as good a job as possible with your patients? What kind of feedback do you use to gauge how well you're doing? What are you focusing on currently to try to do a better job? If you need help in this area, let me know how we can help you.

- The federal government now requires patient satisfaction measurement and reporting for hospitals and large clinical groups. In the future, it will be required for most practice settings. We intend to comply with regulatory standards.

Objections to better patient engagement are prevalent and popular in certain circles. The number of shares of the KevinMD blog posting underscores that point. Some objections are based on logic. Others are born of frustration. Regardless, if a doctor's patient satisfaction scores are low or if he gets complaints from patients, he needs to get past his objections and get on board with figuring out how to do better.

I'm Not a Natural at Interacting with Patients (I'm Kind of a Nerd)

Some physicians were born with the ability to relate well with patients, and yes, they do have an advantage. But many others have evolved from Dr. Aloof or Dr. Awkward to Dr. Personable because they worked at it.

Think about this:

- As much as relating to patients is an art, it is also a science. An interaction can be broken into key parts that occur nearly every time. These components can be learned—practiced, improved on, and eventually mastered.
- The single biggest factor that helps in this transition is simply being mindful of the importance of each interaction. Just thinking about it will improve performance. Consider what happened in the First Physician Corporation case study discussed in Chapter 8: Scores began to improve as soon as the group began talking about the issue.
- Some proven approaches for introverts to become better at interacting with their patients include
  - repeating back key information,
  - summarizing key points of the exchange,
  - making sure patients understand how you arrive at your clinical conclusions,
  - asking patients if your conclusion makes sense to them, and
  - always asking if patients have questions before you leave.

Over time, these approaches will become internalized and a natural part of your routine.

I'm Too Busy to Focus on This

The problem here is overcoming McChesney, Covey, and Huling's (2012) so-called whirlwind—the overwhelming crush of issues and tasks that you deal with just to get through a normal workday. The whirlwind sucks up every available minute, leaving zero time to focus on improving.

Try this:

- As we've emphasized throughout the book, choose one new behavior to work on. It should be the *single biggest opportunity* you have to improve your interactions with patients. If you focus on one very important thing, you can make it happen even inside the whirlwind. It may take weeks or a month to master it, but it will happen.

Why Pick on Me? The People at the Front Desk Are Rude!

It's OK that deflection and blame are so hardwired into human nature, because it's among the easiest objections to address.

Here's how I respond:

- I agree—the folks at the front desk need to do better. But that's a different conversation. Remember, it's the patients' interaction with you that trumps all other experiences during their visit. Your efforts have magnified importance to them.
- You don't have to be so incredible that your patients' interaction with you dissolves their dissatisfaction with other aspects of the system. You just have to do a good job with *your* interaction with patients. That's all, and that's something you can control.

Clinical Care Is My Priority

This is the noblest of objections—but it still poses a barrier to providing the best possible care and becoming "my wonderful doctor" in the eyes of your patients.

The healthiest perspective balances multiple priorities, such as providing good clinical care, treating patients (and other members of the team) right, and being productive. The key is to understand that several priorities always merit your attention.

Consider this:

- Doctors who are exceptional clinicians sometimes lose patients to other (not nearly as technically skilled) providers, just because the other doctors are more pleasant to deal with.
- The doctor–patient relationship is exceptionally intimate, in its way, and involves caring not only for the body but also for the soul, mind, and spirit. So the "soft" elements of care are very important. These include anticipating questions before they're asked, helping patients make sense of complicated information, and putting patients at ease.

- Patients who have good relationships with their doctors don't want to disappoint them. This sentiment leads to greater compliance, which leads to better clinical outcomes—it's all related.

Most doctors are bright, logical people. Even if you occasionally find yourself jumping to one of these objections, I hope you catch yourself doing it and consider a different point of view that will result in addressing the issue and improving your scores.

REFERENCES

BirdStrike, MD. 2013. "The Focus on Patient Satisfaction Is Enough to Make You Sick." Kevin MD.com. Published November 19. www.kevinmd.com/blog/2013/11/focus-patient-satisfaction-sick.html.

McChesney, C., S. Covey, and J. Huling. 2012. *The 4 Disciplines of Execution: Achieving Your Wildly Important Goals.* New York: Free Press.

Part V

ADDITIONAL ADVICE SPECIFIC TO SPECIALTY OR PRACTICE SETTING

CHAPTER 11

Advice for Emergency Medicine Physicians and Urgent Care Providers

THIS CHAPTER (as well as chapters 12 and 13) expands on the nuts-and-bolts advice offered in Chapter 1 by offering insights specific to specialty and practice setting. You might find it helpful to revisit Chapter 1 before you read this part of the book, or flip back to that chapter as you continue reading.

ADVICE FOR EMERGENCY MEDICINE PHYSICIANS

Building Rapport with First Impressions

Making a great first impression with a patient and building rapport quickly is important for emergency medicine doctors because you often don't have a history with your patients and your relationship is brief. So it will be worth your time to squeeze all the relationship-building behavior you can into those first few minutes with a patient.

Being Conscious of Body Position

Whether you sit or stand, be intentional about making your patient feel as comfortable as possible in the interaction.

The general advice to sit when talking with a patient is overstated, in my opinion. Instead, sit or stand at a distance that seems appropriate and doesn't cause difficulty for the patient to see and converse with you. Adjust your position if you sense any discomfort from the patient as he holds his head up to speak with you, especially if he is lying on a stretcher.

Keep in mind that standing at the end of the bed can make you seem distant, both literally and figuratively. On the other hand, don't hover over the patient, invading his space, unless you're examining him.

Ensuring Privacy

Privacy is always an issue in the emergency department (ED), especially if you're working in cubicles with curtains. Help protect your patient's privacy, and get credit for doing it.

- If your ED doesn't have individual patient rooms with solid doors, make sure to draw the patient's curtain before you talk—and mention why you're doing it so that you get credit for paying attention to her needs:

  There's a lot going on in the ER today! Let me just close this curtain so you'll have more privacy.

- Be conscious of the volume of your speaking voice. One way that ED patients and their families pass the time is by listening in on conversations in the next cubicle. Reduce those opportunities if possible.

Helping the Patient Understand What to Expect from the ED

Many patients don't understand the role of the ED. Some people use the ED in lieu of primary care. Others expect the ED to completely resolve the issue they present with. Most expect the ED to help relieve their anxiety.

I'm not advocating that you give an educational speech to every patient on exactly what the ED can and can't do for them. I *am* recommending that you be aware of situations where patients are expecting something the ED just doesn't deliver. In those cases, you can provide some background to help patients recalibrate their expectations:

  Our job is to assess you, do what can be done to address your immediate medical needs, and refer you to the appropriate care setting for further care if needed. If we don't think it's safe for you to go home, we can admit you to the hospital. Other times, we refer patients to their primary care doctor or another specialist. Sometimes we can treat your issue here without further follow-up.

Validating Their Decision to Come In

Most patients come to the ED because they are anxious about their health. They will not have made that decision lightly. Most will have asked themselves, "Is this condition serious enough that I interrupt my day/night and sit and wait to be seen?" "Is my situation serious enough that I go and bother the ER doctors?"

So even when they aren't seriously ill, if you think they deserve the benefit of the doubt (and most patients do), reassure them that they made the right decision:

> I can understand why you came in. Our job is to get a handle on what's going on with you. Then we can make good decisions about the best way to proceed. We will take good care of you.

The First Physician Corporation (FPC) emergency doctors (see the case study in Chapter 8) made a fundamental shift in how they viewed nonemergent patients. Brian Tsang, MD, FPC president, says:

> We had to reset our thinking as emergency medicine [EM] providers. As EM doctors we like to treat critically ill patients. But most ED patients aren't very sick. In fact, most have non-life-threatening conditions, but the symptoms have made them so worried that something terrible is happening, that their fear and anxiety actually become their most acute problems.
>
> The fact is that we never thought our noncritical patients needed much of our attention. We also felt powerless to help them if they did not have a treatable acute diagnosis. Once we knew that a patient wasn't seriously ill, we mentally moved on to the next patient, hoping they might have a problem that we could actually fix.
>
> We needed to change that mind-set. We needed to see ourselves as caring for not just a few critical patients, but for an entire community, and embrace the noncritical patients as just as important as anyone else. We needed to understand that even if there was no treatable emergency, these patients needed something from us, that we could provide that something, and that they would appreciate our help just as much [as] or more than the patient we had just resuscitated in the next room.
>
> Our thinking matured so that we understood that satisfying our noncritical patients was not really that hard. It just required a shift in focus—away from the ABCs and critical actions, and toward active listening, empathy, connection, and validation. It doesn't take that much more time, but it does require investing more of our real selves (as opposed to our doctor selves) in patient interactions. The unexpected benefit is that this approach turns

potentially frustrating patient interactions into positive ones and makes the job more rewarding overall.

Communicating During the Physical Exam

Patients take the physical exam seriously. Multitasking in the form of asking questions during the exam gives the impression that you aren't paying attention to what you could be learning from your inspection.

My advice: Instead of asking questions, report to the patient what you're finding as you palpate and listen. Even something as simple as "no swelling in the lymph nodes" is appreciated by the patient.

Managing Handoffs to Hospitalists or at Shift Change

In care transitions, patients have to trade the relationship they've built with you for a new one with an unknown doctor. They're wondering, "Who's behind door number 2?" To minimize the patient's unease at handoff, take the following steps:

- Always let a patient hear from you directly whether she is being admitted. Explain why admission is the right course of action for her. She will especially appreciate you citing a concern for her safety along with other clinical reasoning. Explain that another doctor will be taking care of her once she's admitted. Furthermore, explain what admission is (not everyone knows) and say explicitly that you have informed the new doctor about her case:

    Given X, Y and Z, I think it's best that we admit you overnight because _____. Getting a bed ready can take a while, so bear with us. The team is looking for an open bed right now.

    Getting admitted also means another doctor will be taking care of you up there. [If known:] Today, that will be Dr. Smith. She is a hospitalist, which means she specializes in taking care of patients while they are in the hospital. I've talked with her already. She'll have access to all the test results we've run and all the notes I've made in your medical record.

    Do you have any questions for me about getting admitted to the hospital?

    Ok. We'll try to keep you updated while they're getting that bed ready.

Ideally, you will stop back to see the patient one more time before she goes so that you can say goodbye and give her your best wishes:

I probably won't see you again, so I wanted to say goodbye and wish you well. I've enjoyed meeting you. I wish it could have been under better circumstances.

- If you have to transition a patient's care to another member of your group at shift change, refer to the doctor who will follow you as your "partner" or "colleague" and give the patient the doctor's name if you know it.

  Using the terms *partner* and *colleague* implies that you know and trust the other doctor, which will give the next physician a head start in building a relationship with the patient. The patient will feel more confident knowing she is being cared for by a cohesive team.

Acknowledging Pain

Helping patients deal with pain is a standard of care. Although it's not my job to advise you on that, I've noticed that some physicians do a much better job with pain in the eyes of their patients by

- making sure patients understand that dealing with their pain is a priority,
- letting patients know about how long it takes for the medication to begin working, and
- asking them how the medication is working after it has been administered.

Dealing with Drug Seekers

As mentioned earlier in the book, the ED attracts more of these types of patients than any other healthcare setting does. I consider drug seekers to be patients and customers (so they need to be treated with respect) but also as manipulators (so they deserve a special approach). It's worth repeating here how to deal with drug-seeking behavior using a kind yet straightforward approach:

My concern is that those drugs are very addictive and they could easily harm you. I'd like to refer you to a pain specialist who can help you with your discomfort.

Most drug seekers don't want to have anything to do with a pain specialist, and they tend to know you're on to them when you suggest this.

Because dealing with drug seekers is such a difficult and pervasive issue, consider working with the other physicians and care providers in your group to develop best-practice responses to be used by all.

Using Images When You Can

In Chapter 1, I recommended "showing your work." This means sharing your clinical thinking with patients so that they can more clearly understand and buy into your conclusions. One way to do this in the ED is to print out a copy of any image taken and show it to the patient and his family. As with the physical exam, showing a relevant image calls on more of the patient's senses. It demonstrates the thoroughness of your work and may help the patient more fully understand his situation.

Addressing Wait Times

A big dissatisfier for patients in the ED is waiting, but waiting is usually unavoidable. Even if you could clone yourself, there are many causes of long wait times outside of your control. Acknowledging waits and setting expectations will go a long way toward diffusing patient unhappiness.

- When you finally see a patient who has been waiting a long time, address the delay head on, using the AAA approach from Chapter 1: Acknowledge, Apologize, Amend. This approach helps assuage the patient's frustration and lets her be more fully present for her interaction with you now that it is finally happening. It will move her focus from "the wait" to "my treatment."

- Keep in mind that the patient's *perception* of his wait time is more important to his satisfaction than the *actual* wait time he experiences. Having no idea how long something may take always makes the wait *feel* longer. Give the patient a sense of how long a step in his care may take so that he can calibrate his expectations: *"Sometimes it can take an hour to get those lab results back."* Take care not to overpromise and underdeliver. Sometimes you might simply have to say that the wait may be long and you can't accurately estimate how long it will be. Even this is helpful, because it shows that you are aware and care, and it helps the patient adjust his expectations.

- If you know a patient has been waiting a long time for test results, use a quick "middle visit" to show her you know she's still there:

  We're still waiting on those labs results. As soon as I get them, I'll be in to go over them with you. Are you still doing OK?

- If you can spare 30 seconds for a middle visit, you can make a tremendous impression:

  It took a while to get through this visit, but my doctor never forgot about me. He truly cares! What a great human being.

Preventing Discharge Anxiety

A quick repeat of three key tips from Chapter 1 is in order here:

1. Make sure you review discharge instructions as you wrap things up and say goodbye to the patient, and remember to tell the patient that instructions will also be given by the nurse and again in writing.
2. Remember that most patients come to the ED because they are anxious about their immediate health. This anxiety may still be present when it is time to discharge them home, especially in the following situations:
   – Cases that were borderline admissions, but you decided against admitting the patient
   – Cases in which patients think they should have been admitted, but that action clearly was not indicated
   – Cases in which patients expected you to completely resolve their problem, but now they'll have to rely on an office-based doctor to do that

     Doctors who excel at handling these situations also explain why it's safe to go home and what type of occurrence might make a return to the ED a good option (recognizing that, ultimately, the patient will be the judge of that): *"Please don't hesitate to return if you ever feel afraid due to your health"* is a nice way to wrap up. One of the biggest ways you help your patients is by giving them peace of mind.
3. Say goodbye. Doctors who fail to do this miss a major opportunity to cement their patients' positive impression of them in their minds. My clients often tell me how pleasantly surprised patients seem when they stop in to say a heartfelt goodbye and to wish them well.

ADVICE FOR URGENT CARE PROVIDERS

Most of the advice from Chapter 1 applies to providers in an urgent care setting, but I've seen additional specific issues pop up repeatedly for my urgent care clients.

Explaining Your Role if You're a Physician's Assistant or a Nurse Practitioner

If you're a mid-level healthcare provider—a physician's assistant (PA) or a nurse practitioner (NP)—how, when, and what do you communicate about your role to a patient who expects to be seen by a physician or who doesn't understand what you do? Do you deal with this proactively, or do you wait to see if the patient raises the issue? This question can be surprisingly tricky to answer.

If you bring it up when you first meet every patient, you may be making a big deal out of nothing for someone who *doesn't* have questions about your role, and then you run the risk of sounding defensive. But if you wait for the patient to raise a question, you leave the issue unaddressed for someone who isn't comfortable bringing it up.

I don't have a perfect answer, but here are some ideas to help guide you in these situations:

- Regardless of whether you take the proactive or wait-and-see approach, have literature available that explains your role.
- Ask another member of the urgent care team, such as the medical assistant, to introduce you:

  Ms. Carter will be in to see you shortly. She's a physician's assistant. If you've never been seen by a PA before, they are trained and licensed to treat the straightforward ailments and conditions we treat in our urgent care center. If you have any questions, here is a brochure, or you can ask her. She's an excellent clinician.

- Address the issue yourself with every patient at the beginning of your encounter:

  Hello, I'm Nancy Smith. I'm a physician's assistant, and I'll be taking care of you today. If you're not familiar with PAs, I'm trained and licensed to handle the straightforward ailments and conditions we treat in our urgent care center, like your sore throat. If we happen to discover something more serious today, I will refer you to the ER right away.

- If you prefer to wait and respond to questions if they're asked, make sure your sixth sense is attuned to those that go unraised.

Avoiding Unexplained Absences

I see this again and again in urgent care settings, especially from introverted clients: The provider has to leave the room—often to get supplies—but doesn't tell the patient why.

You know where you're going and why, but the patient has no clue: *"Did the PA forget about me? Is she taking care of someone else now? Is she coming back?"* All it takes to preempt this anxiety is a simple, *"I'll be right back. I have to get some supplies."*

Preventing Discharge Anxiety

Sometimes, fairly complex discharge instructions are given in urgent care. Because the patient is often not referred to another provider for follow-up, the stakes for compliance can be high. To help your patients feel less anxious about "getting it right" (and to help ensure that they do), review the discharge tips provided earlier in the "Advice for Emergency Medicine Physicians" section.

CHAPTER 12

Advice for Hospitalists (and Other Providers Who Round on Inpatients)

THIS CHAPTER EXPANDS on the more general advice offered in Chapter 1 by addressing opportunities for improving patient satisfaction in the inpatient setting. The tips that follow are specifically intended for hospitalists, but many could apply to any specialist providing care to inpatients.

EASING THE TRANSITION TO INPATIENT STATUS

When patients are admitted, most frequently after spending time in the emergency department, they are making a significant transition to a new setting with a new care team. And they have to build relationships and trust with a new physician—or, more likely, physicians—unless their stay is very short or the hospital is very small. If you are the first hospitalist the patient sees after admission, you can help her through this process by taking the following approach:

- Reemphasize that these changes are in her best interest.
- Make sure she understands why she is being admitted, and emphasize that an inpatient unit is the safest place for her to be.
- Review findings from her history, physical exam, and tests.
- Set expectations early for her likely plan of treatment, any additional tests that will be completed, and any consultants she should expect to see during her hospital stay.

All this information may have been delivered an hour before by the emergency medicine physician. That's OK; patients and families usually need to hear information more than once for the key points to fully sink in, especially when they are scared, sick, and overwhelmed. And patients appreciate knowing the new physician is fully up to speed on the important facts regarding their care. Continuity of care is important to patients.

ARTICULATING WHAT HOSPITALISTS DO

Many hospitalists have found that taking the time to clearly and accurately explain their role is worth the effort, especially for newly admitted patients. Hospitalist medicine is a relatively new specialty, and most people still don't get it. Sell yourself and your partners, and ease the patient's anxiety, with an introduction such as this:

> I am a hospitalist. Caring for hospital patients has become increasingly complex, so now there are doctors who specialize in it, just like your personal doctor specializes in caring for you in her office. So my partners and I will manage your care as you are admitted and during your hospital stay. One of us will be available for you 24 hours a day while you are here. We will bring in other specialists to help if they are needed, but *we are the "captains of your ship."* Do you have any questions about that?

Following are some additional guidelines for helping inpatients understand the hospitalist role:

- One exceptional hospital I've worked with prints the definition of *hospitalist* in lay terms on the back of its hospitalists' business cards.
- Better still, some hospitals produce a brochure that introduces your practice and explains what hospitalists do. Provide copies for patients and their families to look at later.
- If physicians outside your hospitalist group will be cycling through their room, patients will be grateful if you take a moment to explain their roles as well. In a perfect world, each provider will introduce himself and explain how his job fits into the larger picture of the care team, but that doesn't always happen. (And even when it does, patients may not understand until they've heard an explanation several times.) This is *not* what you want your patients to feel:

> Why are there so many different doctors? Do they talk to each other? Do they even know about each other? Are they duplicating each other's

efforts? Are they unwittingly doing things that screw up other things? *Do they all know what's going on with me?*

- Make it clear that you and your hospitalist partners are in regular communication with the patient's other specialists. Give the patient faith that someone—you—is coordinating it all.

USING BUSINESS CARDS

All the advice from Chapter 1 about making a good first impression on patients also applies to hospitalists, of course. But after watching some excellent hospitalists in action, I want to emphasize how significantly a business card can add value:

- Get into the practice of leaving your business card, especially if patients or family members have asked a lot of questions—or you sense they might later. Consider it a communications safety net as well as a kind gesture. Remember that when patients communicate well with you, they are helping you provide excellent medical care.
- Some doctors hand out their cards immediately upon introducing themselves, but it tends to carry greater impact as the physician says goodbye at the end of that first interaction: *"Here's my card; please contact me if you have any questions."* If you give it earlier in the visit, it can get lost in the craziness of introductions and getting started.
- Some of the most effective business cards include the physician's picture. (These can be black and white pictures—no expensive color printing necessary.) Patients and families may meet several hospitalists from your practice during their stay. The picture will help them keep track of who's who.

HANDING OFF TO ANOTHER HOSPITALIST

If you are taking a few days off and your patients will be seeing a different doctor from your group tomorrow, let them know this. As I've mentioned earlier in the book, I recommend referring to the doctor whom the patients will see tomorrow as your "partner" or "colleague," and use your colleague's name if you know who it will be. Even if you can't provide a name, using these terms gives a better impression than saying "another doctor" will be taking over.

It may be helpful to let your patients know that tomorrow's doctor may ask some questions that they have already answered. Assure them that the doctor will have a full report on their case and that the questions are just to be sure the doctor has the story right.

- It seems obvious, but it bears mentioning: Never criticize other hospitalists, specialists, or primary care physicians (PCPs) in front of your patients. When a doctor wonders out loud, "Why did she do that?" patients almost always interpret this as criticism of the other provider. The result: Anxiety and an instant and significant loss of trust in the care team.

REMEMBERING YOUR VISIT IS THE PATIENT'S DAILY HIGHLIGHT

Although it's just another stop on your busy schedule, your visit with a patient—especially one whose stay is lengthy—is the highlight of her day. The rest of the time is just waiting around for your appearance! Family members may have even arranged their work schedules to have the best shot at being present when you show up. Following are ways you can demonstrate that you take this time together seriously:

- Before each visit, pause and recognize the importance of the visit for the patient and her family. Vow not to "short" them, even if there's not much news to relay that day. That doesn't mean you have to stay for an extended chitchat. But make sure to give the visit the time necessary to cover all the important business and fully answer questions. As I'm sure you're aware, families sitting in hospital rooms with time on their hands tend to come up with lots of new questions.
- It may help to have an agenda for each visit and share it with the patient right away: *"Today we're going to talk about how you're doing, go over the results of the tests we ran yesterday, and discuss when you might be going home."* Recognize that hospitalized patients are often anxious about the results of every test—even those you view as mundane. I've seen superstar doctors go the extra mile by visiting the patient a second time in the same day to report the results of "high stakes" tests. Some exemplary physicians go a step or two further; read the experiences of two such hospitalists in the sidebar.
- Make a tremendously positive impression by asking, *"Is there anything else that I can do for you today?"* right before you leave the room. Something as simple as adjusting the room temperature sends the message, *"Wow, my doctor really cares about me."*

Two Physicians Share Their Advice on Patient Communications

Ana Laus, MD, a hospitalist at St. Luke's Hospital in New Bedford, Massachusetts, has achieved exemplary patient satisfaction scores by taking her communications with patients' families one step further (personal communication, March 10, 2015):

> Recently I've gotten into the practice of offering to call family members if no one is present in the patient's room during rounds. Patients are usually overwhelmed about their condition, sometimes they are forgetful, sometimes they cannot keep track of "who is who" with so many professionals involved with their care (physicians, nurses, technicians, phlebotomists, respiratory therapists, etc.).

> Even if the patient is competent to make his or her own decisions, I find that the vast majority always want me to contact a relative to discuss their condition and plan of care (children, spouse, healthcare proxy, etc.). Of course, consent needs to be given before contacting a third party due to HIPAA [Health Insurance Portability and Accountability Act] rules.

This is a great practice, in my opinion. When the family members arrive at the hospital, they already know what the plan of care that day is for the patient. By keeping families well informed, you have more satisfied clients. It may even save you a few pages later in the day, because when relatives arrive at the hospital at a later time, they already know what is going on. . . . And many times, these family members are the ones who will be filling out the patient satisfaction questionnaire later on.

Jamie Witkowski, MD, of Charlton Memorial Hospital in Fall River, Massachusetts, reports similar positive results (personal communication, March 28, 2015):

> Taking an extra few minutes to call a designated family member every day goes a long way in helping the patient and family to gain trust in me. Sometimes I have to force myself to do it because it can be tedious and it's easy to blow off. But afterwards I am usually very glad I made the call.

USING THE WHITEBOARD TO REINFORCE COMMUNICATIONS

Sometimes I've heard patients say that their doctor didn't keep them informed, when what really happened is that the doctor didn't keep them informed *enough*. As I've mentioned before, patients often need to hear things several times before they absorb the information. Many hospitals now provide whiteboards in patient rooms, and these boards are a great tool for making sure patients (and family members) "hear" your message again and again. Here are a few tips for using whiteboards effectively:

- Use the board to quickly note a plan for the patient every day, including any major tests or procedures scheduled or test results expected. Even if the plan is just that the patient rests and gets stronger that day, note it: *"Regain strength."* This note acts like a prescription—a specific, well-considered course of treatment that the patient perceives as an act of healing; he's not just lying there "doing nothing."
- Write legibly!

ANSWERING THE PATIENT'S BIGGEST QUESTION

"When will I get discharged?" Whether patients want to go home ASAP or are scared they'll be discharged too soon, this is the biggest question—voiced or unvoiced—that patients have throughout their stay. Address the ever-present query with the following in mind:

- Each day, continue to state what is keeping the patient in the hospital and where his status needs to progress before discharge can be considered. Remember, your brain is trained to think about this automatically, but the patient needs to hear what you're thinking, and he probably needs to hear it more than once.
- The patient and his family feel most secure when the messages they receive from doctors, nurses, and other providers are consistent. Inconsistencies in communication make the patient worry that there may be inconsistencies in clinical care: *"Do they all really know what's going on with my treatment? Where else is the ball getting dropped?"*

Seek to do an exceptional job of making sure to discuss the plan of care daily not only with the patient but also with the case managers and nursing staff. If you're lucky, you work for a hospital that conducts brief, daily multidisciplinary rounds where all involved providers discuss the care for each patient. If not, you could help champion adoption of this model.

COORDINATING WITH THE PRIMARY CARE PHYSICIAN

You know that communicating with the patient's PCP can lead to better care because you may learn new information about the patient. But did you know that you also get bonus points in the trust department when you *tell the patient* you've talked with her personal physician?

Jamie Witkowski, MD (see sidebar) makes sure all of his patients know that he will communicate with their PCP about major issues, and he reassures patients that their PCP will receive a full report of everything that is done at the hospital. To solidify their trust in the continuity of care, he goes an extraordinary extra mile:

> I have tried to get to know the local PCPs on a personal level so that I can relate a personal anecdote that conveys to the patient that I know their PCP.

CHAPTER 13

Advice for Primary Care Providers (and Other Providers Who See Patients in an Office Setting)

WHEN IT COMES to satisfying and engaging patients, primary care physicians have an advantage that other specialties do not: the opportunity to build relationships with patients over years and years. But every primary care colleague has this advantage. How will you distinguish yourself when it comes to interacting with your patients? Here are some tips especially for you.

AVOIDING THE IMPRESSION YOU'RE IN A RUSH

"Not enough time with my doctor" is a leading reason patients are not satisfied with their care. But there's no magic amount of time that you must spend with each patient, and most will respect your need to keep moving. Here are two keys to leaving your patients satisfied with the amount of time you're able to spend with them:

1. Don't send unintended (or, heaven forbid, intended) signals that you have more important things to do. Be totally immersed in serving each patient during the time you're with him. Be conscious of body language that says otherwise. Don't check your watch or pager. Sit down, if that's comfortable for you, even if just for a minute or two. Maintain eye contact and be an active listener.

    Peter Baldwin, MD, a family practice physician in Dayton, Ohio, takes special care as he accesses the patient's electronic health record during visits (personal communication, April 2, 2015): "A computer can sometimes be in the way. I consider the room setup and the placement of keyboards and monitors. And I explain to patients that I'm writing some notes about their care."

2. Avoid "shorting" the patient by seeming annoyed with his questions or cutting him off as he's telling his story. (Of course, you have to exercise some judgment on this point if a patient wants to talk about tangential matters forever. See the "Dealing with the *War and Peace* Recitations" section later in this chapter for handling these occasions.)

ENCOURAGING GOOD QUESTIONS—YOURS AND THEIRS

A comfortable exchange of information between patient and doctor is critical if the patient is to feel his needs were met. Asking for questions at the end of the visit is an important but *minimum* requirement. The doctors with the happiest patients adopt a more thorough and thoughtful approach:

- I'll start with the obvious: Never treat patients' questions dismissively. Doing so will damage their willingness to ask other (maybe very important) questions later.

- Be aware that some patients won't ask all the questions they have. Become attuned to that reluctance; your sixth sense will begin to tell you when they're holding back. You might help them ask the unasked question by saying, *"Sometimes my patients with your condition are curious about _____."*

- Other patients will muster up the courage to mention another reason (maybe the real reason) for their visit only when your hand is on the doorknob to leave. When that happens, turn around, sit back down, or otherwise "reenter" the conversation. Preface whatever you say next with, *"I'm glad you asked about that,"* if appropriate.

PLUSSES AND MINUSES TO MULTITASKING

Do you try to multitask and ask questions during the physical exam? Some of my clients do this very well, and it makes them more productive. Others send the (unintended) message that they are giving sufficient attention to neither exercise! Consider the following thoughts on the topic:

- If you're new at it, acknowledge you're attempting double duty: *"May I ask you some more questions while I'm examining you?"* Be sure to state afterward that everything looked fine on the physical exam so that the patient knows you were taking it seriously.

- It's helpful to describe what you're doing through all parts of the exam, especially with pediatric patients.
- If you struggle with this multitasking or are unsure of the message you may be sending by asking questions during the exam, ask someone you trust to watch you and give you her opinion.

OFFERING REASSURANCE ALONGSIDE YOUR GREETING

Primary care doctors often handle greetings a bit differently than specialists or other types of providers do because they have ongoing relationships with their patients. Following are some key points for this exchange:

- In your greeting, demonstrate that you remember patients with a simple, *"Hi. It's good to see you again!"* Ideally, you'll develop a system in your chart to help prompt you with some personal information on each patient that you can reference to build rapport. Minimally, you'll have clinical information from prior visits you can mention to underscore the ongoing nature of your relationship.
- Reassure patients that they made a good choice to come see you about their medical issues (even for well-patient visits). Patients want a supportive doctor. So help them feel like they made a good decision: *"I'm glad you decided to come in. We're going to figure this out and, I hope, get you feeling better."*

Maybe you can't do much about her cold virus, but your patient will see you are a caring partner in her healthcare. The next time she needs a doctor, she'll call you again.

PLACING PARAMETERS ON THE VISIT

You've undoubtedly encountered patients who schedule an appointment to address problem X but ask you to also deal with Y and Z once they've arrived. This puts you in a difficult position. Many doctors try to accommodate patients to the extent possible. But when it's not feasible to do so, this kind of statement may work as a diplomatic way to handle the situation:

It looks like you have more concerns than we knew about when we set up the appointment. And we only scheduled enough time today to address your _____. I think the most important problem to deal with today is the _____. But let me do this for your other issues: We'll schedule a follow-up appointment so that we can give them the time they deserve. And I'll recommend some over-the-counter remedies to ease your discomfort until we meet to address those issues.

If you practice in a group, I recommend spending some time together discussing how others deal with this tricky issue. There are bound to be some clever best practices among your colleagues.

DEALING WITH THE *WAR AND PEACE* RECITATIONS

One of the skills I most value in any person is an ability to communicate the key points of a complex situation completely yet succinctly. However, many patients lack this skill, and some take every available tangent out for a test drive. Applying diplomacy in these situations is a huge challenge for primary care physicians. Some ideas to deal with this situation are as follows:

- When it's apparent that the patient won't stop on her own and she's adding no information of value, it's OK to interrupt. But interrupt as gently as you can: *"I see. Let me jump in here. You're giving me a lot of information, but is there anything else you can tell me that relates to [the medical condition]?"* Or, *"I hear what you're saying about A, B, and C, but I don't think those are related to [the medical condition]. Is there anything more to add that might be related to that?"*
- If the patient responds apologetically or defensively, add something like, *"Think nothing of it. Sometimes patients can't be sure if information is related or not. It's my job to let you know."*
- Remember, you can always switch over to closed-ended questions to navigate the situation. Breaking in with a simple, *"I see. Does your throat hurt?"* can interrupt a flow of mostly irrelevant information and allow you to gain control.

MAKING REFERRALS

If you need to refer your patient to a specialist or clinic, remember that this is a major event for her. She must leave the comfortable, trusting relationship she has built with you to see a new caregiver, and on top of that, it's often for a new or significant health concern. Ease this transition by using the following tactics:

- Emphasize the expertise she will receive from the specialist and why you think getting that expertise is important for her health.
- Offer her choices in specialists when possible. Check to see if she has a preference.
- Reassure her that you will remain her personal physician: *"You'll probably continue to see that group for _____ care, but I will continue to be your doctor for other things. We'll share information back and forth with their office as necessary. Does that sound reasonable? May we make that referral for you?"*
- If you need to refer your patient to a specialist or clinic, be very specific about who *you think* will be calling whom to set up the appointment, when that might happen, and so on. Of course you can't make promises related to the operations of another practice, but merely telling your patient "We're going to send you to a cardiologist" does nothing to relieve her anxiety. To the extent you can, proactively address the referral logistics, or make sure your assistant does.

Baldwin goes one step further and sets up a follow-up visit with patients after they've seen the specialist. "That way, I can hear the patient's interpretation of the specialist's findings and compare it to the specialist's note. I have the opportunity to interpret the plan for them or answer any questions that may have arisen in the interim."

COMMUNICATING ABOUT TESTS

Waiting for any but the most mundane test results can be worrisome for your patients. They will appreciate it if you take the time to make sure they know what the name of the test is, what it's for, how it will be administered (Will there be discomfort? Will it take long?), when results should be available, and how results will be communicated (or not communicated—when results are normal, for example).

Waiting for results of a high-stakes test is a time of high stress for patients. Let them know how long it can take to get those results and what they can do to speed the process along: *"If you haven't heard from us about the results within three days, please don't hesitate to give us a call."*

INVITING RE-CLOTHING

I see this problem again and again: As the doctor is completing the visit, he fails to let the patient know it's OK—once the doctor exits—to put his pants back on. Don't make your patient wait for the nurse to give him permission. Remember, you know the routine but your patient does not. Patients want to get dressed ASAP, and you'll score extra points when you give them the green light to go ahead and do it. (And in the process, you'll help turn over the room more quickly.)

ADDRESSING ANTIBIOTICS REQUESTS

Patients insisting on an antibiotics prescription for a cold virus is a sticky wicket for doctors everywhere. You want to serve your patient, but you need to respect the science of medicine. I have two suggestions:

1. Have discussions with your colleagues to develop best-practice approaches for how to deal with this request. The collective wisdom of the group can benefit all its members.

2. Until you establish a best-practice approach in your group, try saying this:

    You've tested negative for a bacterial infection. That means antibiotics won't help you. And prescribing antibiotics when you don't need them helps "superbugs" become resistant to antibiotics, which could be serious for anyone who might get them—including you. Most viruses go away on their own. I can tell you about ways to treat the symptoms of your virus that are making you feel cruddy. If the symptoms don't clear up in X days, we'll get you back in to test for a bacterial infection. Does that seem reasonable?

A Final Word

I WANT YOU to be a superstar in the eyes of your patients. Your patients want you to be a superstar, too.

The fact that you've made it this far in this book shows that you're thinking you might have opportunities to improve—and that you are willing to think about changing some behaviors to make an impact on how much your patients appreciate you.

Congratulations! Taking a little time to thoughtfully focus on improving is something very few people do. It is too easy to get absorbed into the drama of the moment or the fire that needs fighting now and never get around to improving.

I hope this book gives you practical insight on what to do next. A few things to remember:

- Every three or four months, take a look at your patient satisfaction survey scores and verbatim comments from patients. These will help you track your progress from 30,000 feet.

- Have a game plan that details issues you could work on to have better interactions with your patients. Chapters 1, 11, 12, and 13 offer plenty of ideas, and the tools in Chapter 5 will help you identify behaviors that will have the most impact for you.

- Work on one behavior change at a time: Try something new, see how it goes, adjust, try it again, and so on—until you're performing it every time without thinking about it. This can take a month or even longer. Only then should you move on to the next change.

- Figure out how to keep your current "one change" on your radar screen so that you think about it—even for just a few seconds—every day or several times each week. Otherwise, it will get swept away by the whirlwind of your workday. If you can devote just half of a percent of your brain to this effort, you'll end up in a really good place.

- It's OK if the journey from here to there has ups and downs, and perhaps false starts or pauses. Let me repeat: That's OK. The race is won by those who keep trying.

In six to nine months, you'll be well on your way to being a different doctor in the eyes of your patients. They will notice. Those who work around you will notice. People who have access to your patient satisfaction scores will notice. (Be sure that others get to see those scores!)

And you'll feel different about yourself. You'll be a patient satisfaction leader who can inspire others. Perhaps you'll be asked to mentor or be a role model for some of your colleagues. Dare I congratulate you in advance?

I wish you well on your personal journey!

About the Author

Bo Snyder, FACHE, is a healthcare consultant and speaker who has worked side by side with physicians for 30 years. As adviser and coach, he supports their efforts to improve interactions with patients.

Snyder began his career in administrative roles with Bronson Healthcare Group, working with doctors to improve hospital services and their practices. In Snyder's last few years at Bronson, he was deeply involved in efforts that led to the organization's receipt of the Malcolm Baldrige National Quality Award in 2005.

Every aspect of Snyder's professional life is energized and "made real" by working on the front lines with the doctors, nurses, and others who directly help patients. In addition to speaking and shadow coaching physicians to improve patient satisfaction, Snyder volunteers his time as a Baldrige examiner at the national and state levels, trains other examiners, and leads Baldrige teams and site visits.

Snyder is an adjunct professor in the Department of Health Management and Policy at the University of Michigan School of Public Health. He serves on the alumni board there and mentors current students and recent graduates. And he likes to remind people that the University of Michigan has the top-ranked health services management program in the country.

Snyder holds two degrees from the University of Michigan: from the Ross School of Business and from the Department of Health Management and Policy at the School of Public Health. He has a passionate (some say unhealthy) relationship with Michigan football and has missed only one game at the Big House since 1979.

THE AUTHOR WELCOMES YOUR FEEDBACK

One key point I make in this book is that to improve, one must get input on one's strengths and opportunities for improvement. With that information in hand, decisions on what and how to improve can be made.

I am willing to take my own advice.

Please contact me with comments or suggestions. I am most interested in the following:

- Areas of the book that are the most helpful to you
- Suggestions for changes or additions in future editions
- Your personal experiences that can add value to future editions, including volunteering your group to serve as a case study

You can find me at Bo@BoSnyderConsulting.com.